Yoga Sutras of Patanjali

Proper Translation & Chanting

This book contains

- Original Sanskrit Sutras

- English Transliteration

- Proper meaning of each word

- Proper word sequence (Anvaya)

- English translation of each Sutra

- Key to pronunciation

- Audio CDs containing
  - Oral instruction for chanting
  - Uninterrupted chanting

Yoga Sutras of Patanjali, Proper Translation & Chanting

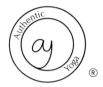

Designed & Printed By:
Akshar Seva
B/4, Keshar Society, B/H Jog Hospital, Paud Road, Pune
Maharashtra 411038. INDIA
Tel.: +91-20-25448173
Email : aksharseva@vsnl.net   Date: July, 2006

Audio CD:
Mastering: Neel Kulkarni
Printing & Replication: Digital Strategies CD Printing Pvt. Ltd.
1378 Shukrawar Peth, Pune 411 002. INDIA
Tel: +91-9422512456, Web: www.digicdp.com

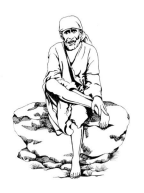

|| श्री साई ||

This book is dedicated to my father, whose association is the cause of all Yoga in me.

It is also dedicated to late N.N. Bhide, my Sanskrit teacher at the New English School, Pune, India. My deepest respects go to Dr. Ganesh Thite, retired Professor and Head of the Department of Sanskrit, Pune University, India, and Pandit Vasantrao Gadgil, founder and editor of Sharada Magazine for Sanskrit. All of these teachers have been a profound inspiration for my lifelong study of Sanskrit and Yoga.

I feel privileged to receive a foreward from Prof. Deviprasad Kharwandikar, renowned Sanskrit Scholar and Poet. In the past, he had also translated my "Health and Yoga Aphorisms" into beautiful Sanskrit verses. As per his suggestion, I plan to prepare and publish a brief commentary on the Sutras.

I must admit that I could not have presented this book without extensive editing and review by my wife, Nancy Kulkarni. I am also thankful to my spiritual sisters, Anne Jablonski and Pam McDonald, for their help in editing this work. The typesetting work done by the staff at Akshar Seva deserves an appreciation from me.

I hope this humble book benefits students of Yoga. Peace and joy!

Neel Kulkarni
Gurupaurnima 2006

Contents

Foreword

I am very happy to introduce Mr. Neel Kulkarni's valuable book on the Yoga-sutras of Patanjali to the students of Yoga. I accepted the task of writing this foreward for two reasons. Firstly, I am a Sanskrit teacher and deeply interested in Indian philosophy. Secondly, I am very much impressed by the studious approach of the author of this book, who has a family background of Yogic practices.

A lot of books on Yoga are available in the market. But the present book by Neel Kulkarni has some unique features that clearly bring out its distinctive qualities. Readers shall find a complete Sanskrit text of the Yoga-sutras with their transliteration in Roman script. The author has used an informal scheme of transliteration which is easy to follow. A very faithful rendering of the Yoga-sutras, at once simple and free from ambiguity, will add to the utility of the book. A special point deserves a note: The author has given the meanings of all the word-forms in their sequential order, which will doubtless help readers to follow the text correctly. Additionally, a valuable set of audio CDs is provided along with the book, that will facilitate chanting and learning the text by heart.

Mr. Neel Kulkarni has thus spared no pains in making this book very useful. I encourage him to publish a supplementary compendium that shall contain commentary on the Sutras and a brief survey of Yoga Darshana.

I am thankful to Mr. Kulkarni for giving me the opportunity to say a few words of appreciation about his book, and more importantly, that he has thus inspired me to apply my mind to the subject of Yoga more than before. I conclude with my own Sanskrit verse highlighting the greatness of Patanjali:

(योगदर्शन प्रणेतारं महर्षि-पतञ्जलिं प्रति सादरं वन्दना । श्लोकः वसन्ततिलकावृत्तम् ।)

चेतोत्रपुर्विकसनाय सदा समेषाम्

अष्टाङ्गयोगमिह यः कथयाञ्चकार ।

येनोज्ज्वलोऽन्धतमसे विदधे सुपन्था

वन्दे पतञ्जलि-मुनिं करुणाकरं तम् ॥

(I bow down to the compassionate Sage Patanjali who has explained the eight-fold Yoga for the mental and physical development of all, and who thus prepared a bright and beautiful path in the pitchy darkness of ignorance.)

Ahmednagar, India _____ Dr. D. K. Kharwandikar

Dr. D. K. Kharwandikar (b.1935) (M.A. Sanskrit - Ardhamagadhi, M.A. - Ancient Indian Culture, Ph. D., Kavyateertha, Sangeet Alankar). Retired Professor - Ahmednagar College. School and University prizes, 2 NCERT prizes, 2 All India Radio prizes, 3 Delhi Sanskrit Academy prizes and many other awards. Honoured by Govt. of Maharashtra with the accolade - "SANSKRIT PANDIT". Chief Editor of Sanskrit Quarterly - Ganjarava. A Sanskrit poet - scholar. He has a number of research articles and Sanskrit compositions to his credit.

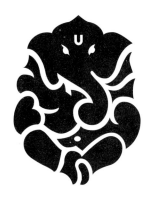

ॐ श्री गणेशाय नमः ।

OM shrii gaNeshaaya namaH

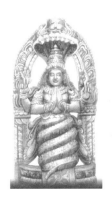

ॐ श्री पतञ्जलये नमः ।

OM shrii pataJNjalaye namaH

योगेन चित्तस्य पदेन वाचाम् ।

मलं शरीरस्य च वैद्यकेन ।

योऽपाकरोत्तं प्रवरं मुनीनाम् ।

पतञ्जलिं प्राञ्जलिरानतोऽस्मि ॥

yogena chittasya padena vaachaaM
malaM shariirasya cha vaidyakena
yo.apaakarottaM pravaraM muniinaaM
pataJNjaliM praaJNjaliraanato.asmi

(Prayer to the sage Patanjali, composed by the famous Sanskrit poet Bhartruhari)

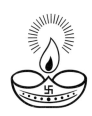

OM. Salutations to Shree Ganesha.　　　　　**OM. Salutations to Shree Patanjali.**

aanato.asmi	I bow down
praaJNjalir	with folded hands
taM	to that
pataJNjaliM	to Patanjali
pravaraM	supreme
muniinaaM	amongst sages
yo	who
apaakarot	removed
malaM	impurity
chittasya	of the Chitta (perceptive faculty of mind)
yogena	by Yoga (that is, Paatanjala Yoga Darshana, a complete, accurate, and most reliable work on Yoga)
yo	who
apaakarot	removed
malaM	impurity
vaachaaM	of communication
padena	by grammer (that is Patanjali Mahaabhaashya, an exhaustive and extremely respected commentary on sage Paanini's Ashtaadhyaayii which is the landmark and standard of Sanskrit grammar)
cha	and
yo	who
apaakarot	removed
malaM	impurity
shariirasya	of body
vaidyakena	by Vaidyaka (that is commentaries on the work of Charaka on Ayurveda, the science of Health)

I bow down with folded hands to Patanjali, the supreme amongst sages, who removed impurity of the Chitta (perceptive faculty of mind) by Yoga (that is, Paatanjala Yoga Darshana, a complete, accurate, and most reliable work on yoga), who removed impurity of communication by grammer (that is Patanjali Mahaabhaashya, an exhaustive and extremely respected commentary on sage Paanini's Ashtaadhyaayii which is the landmark and standard of Sanskrit grammer), and who removed impurity of body by Vaidyaka (that is commentaries on the work of Charaka, a scholar of Ayurveda, the science of Health).

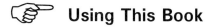 **Using This Book**

• This book is an extremely useful reference for a Yoga philosophy course. Recorded speeches by the translator, Neel Kulkarni, containing a commentary on the Yoga Sutras of Patanjali are also available.

• Knowledge of Sanskrit language, Devanaagari script, and the transliteration scheme used in this book are not essential for understanding the English translation.

• The Sutras must be studied in a sequential order, as the understanding of a particular Sutra is based on the understanding of previous Sutras. Certain Sanskrit terms (such as Yoga, Samaadhi, etc) are used in the translation without definition. These terms are defined by Patanjali himself in the Sutras.

• Those who wish to study the translation of the Sutras without knowing the meaning of each word, should read the fully translated sentences which appears at the end of each Sutra. However, a serious student should strive to understand the meaning of each Sanskrit word.

• Those who know Devanaagari script can read the Sanskrit Sutras. And, others can read the transliteration below each Sanskrit Sutra.

• Those who wish to know the approximate pronunciation of the transliteration should refer to the appendix, which provides a key to pronunciation.

• Those who wish to learn the correct pronunciation of the Sutras should use the Audio CDs (optional) which accompany this book. The CDs provide a format in which the student is given time to repeat the chanting by the teacher. This is followed by uninterrupted chanting which can be studied, contemplated, and used as a background for Yoga exercise practice or meditation.

• The words in the vocabulary list become altered during the chanting. Therefore, proper chanting should be learned from the oral instruction, without use of the vocabulary list.

• A simplified transliteration scheme is presented in the appendix, which provides a key to pronunciation. The words in each vocabulary list are generally given as they appear in the transliterated Sutra, without showing their form before the Sanskrit word-joint (Sandhi). For example see 'yogash' in the Sutra 1:2. In some cases, a word in the vocabulary list may appear with a slight modification due to the peculiarity of Sanskrit. For example, see 'aana.ndaruupa' and 'asmitaaruupa' in Sutra 1:17, and 'smRuti' in Sutra 1:6.

• The Sanskrit words in the English translation are capitalized. For example 'lishavara' from 'iishvara'.

4

Introduction

Yoga Sutras of Patanjali, also called Shree Paatanjala Yoga Darshana, forms a classical work on the subject of Yoga. It was composed by the great sage (Maharshii) Patanjali around 300 B.C., just after the appearance of Gautama Buddha. It contains the entire knowledge of the practical aspect of Yoga. When practiced correctly, Yoga, as described by the sage Patanjali, leads to spiritual liberation called Kaivalya. Although Yoga practice is the main focus of these Sutras, they also include the essential principles of Vedic philosophy. The Paatanjala Yoga Darshana is considered to be the standard text on the Yoga System called Yogadarshana, one of the six systems (Shatdarshana) of the Vedic philosophy.

Understanding the Yoga Sutras of Patanjali requires correct and contextual understanding of each word used in the Sutras. A proper translation of each word is an essential reference for both study and instruction, for students as well as teachers. This book is an attempt in that direction.

Also, the key purpose of composing the entire philosophy into Sutras is for others to memorize and use them at the appropriate time. Memorization is enhanced by chanting the Sutras. Also the chanting provides a great opportunity for contemplation on meaning of the Sutras. Chanting is best learned orally, where the student repeats the chanting by the teacher. The audio CDs which accompany this book provide such an instruction in chanting the Yoga Sutras of Patanjali.

Comprehensive understanding of the Yoga Sutras comes from knowledge of the proper meaning of words used, study of a proper commentary, and sufficient contemplation. Chanting the Sutras enhances the contemplation. Also, chanting has a pleasing and focussing effect on the mind.

In this translation, certain comments are embedded to facilitate understanding. These Sutras encompass a lot of knowledge. Therefore a reasonable understanding of Sutras can only come from study of a commentary. An attempt has been made to keep the original structure of the Sanskrit statements in this translation. It is amazing to study the Yoga Sutras of Patanjali, which present the entire Yoga philosophy in terse, succinct, logical, artistic, and a grammatically interesting form.

अथ श्रीपातञ्जलयोगदर्शनम् - समाधिपादः ।

atha shriipaataJNjalayogadarshanaM samaadhipaadaH

atha	Thus follows
shrii	the divine
yogadarshanaM	treatise on the science of Yoga
paataJNjala	composed by the sage Patanjali
samaadhipaadaH	Chapter Samaadhipaada (which deals with mature stages of meditation)

Thus follows the divine treatise on the science of Yoga composed by the sage Patanjali. This is Chapter Samaadhipaada, which deals with mature stages of meditation.

१. अथ योगानुशासनम् ।

1. atha yogaanushaasanaM

atha	Thus follows
shaasanaM	the science (of)
yoga	Yoga
anu	which came through (the lineage of the Vedas)

Thus follows the science of Yoga which came through the lineage of the Vedas.

२. योगश्चित्तवृत्तिनिरोधः ।

2. yogashchittavRuttinirodhaH

yogash	Yoga (is)
nirodhaH	stoppage (of)
vRutti	(every) modification (of)
chitta	Chitta part of the mental faculty (which deals with perception)

Yoga is stoppage of every modification of Chitta, the part of the mental faculty that deals with perception.

३. तदा द्रष्टुःस्वरूपेऽवस्थानम् ।

3. tadaa drashhTussvaruupe.avasthaanaM

tadaa	Then (When the stoppage of all modifcations is accomplished)
drashhTus	the Seer's (Self of a person)
avasthaanaM	stay
	(occurs)
svaruupe	(only) in its own form

When the stoppage of all modifications is accomplished, the Seer's stay occurs only in its own form.

४. वृत्तिसारूप्यमितरत्र ।
4. vRuttisaaruupyamitaratra

itaratra	elsewhere (At other times, when any modification of the Chitta is present)
saaruupyam	(the Seer's) conformity (occurs)
vRutti	(with that) modification

At other times, that is when any modification of the Chitta is present, the Seer's conformity with that modification occurs.

५. वृत्तयः पञ्चतय्यः क्लिष्टाऽक्लिष्टाः ।
5. vRuttayaH paJNchatayyaH klishhTaa.aklishhTaaH

vRuttayaH	Modifications (of the Chitta are)
paJNchatayyaH	of five kinds
	(and, these five can be either)
klishhTaaH	distressful (or)
aklishhTaaH	non-distressful

Modifications of the Chitta are of five kinds, and these five can be either distressful or non-distressful.

६. प्रमाणविपर्ययविकल्पनिद्रास्मृतयः ।
6. pramaaNaviparyayavikalpanidraasmRutayaH

	(These five modifications are)
pramaaNa	Pramaana
viparyaya	Viparyaya
vikalpa	Vikalpa
nidraa	Nidraa (and)
smRuti	Smruti

These five modifications are Pramaana, Viparyaya, Vikalpa, Nidraa, and Smruti.

७. प्रत्यक्षानुमानागमाः प्रमाणानि ।

7. pratyakshaanumaanaagamaaH pramaaNaani

pramaaNaani	Pramaana modifications (are)
pratyakshaaH	those due to direct perception
anumanaaH	those due to deduction (and)
aagamaaH	those due to reliable sources (such as the Vedas, words or writings of saints, etc.)

Pramaana modifications are due to direct perception, deduction, and reliable sources (such as the Vedas, words or writings of saints, etc.).

८. विपर्ययो मिथ्याज्ञानमतद्रूपप्रतिष्ठम् ।

8. viparyayo mithyaadnyaanamatadruupapratishhThaM

viparyayo	Viparyaya modification (is)
mithyaa	false
dnyaanam	understanding
pratishhThaM	qualified (by)
atadruupa	appearance of a different object (than the perceived one)

Viparyaya modification is a false understanding qualified by the appearance of a different object than the perceived one.

९. शब्दज्ञानानुपाती वस्तुशून्यो विकल्पः ।

9. shabdadnyaanaanupaatii vastushuunyo vikalpaH

vikalpaH	Vikalpa modification (is)
anupaatii	one which is based upon
dnyaana	comprehension (through)
shabda	word(s)
vastushuunyo	where no (actual) object exists

Vikalpa modification is one which is based upon comprehension through words, where no object exists.

१०. अभावप्रत्ययालम्बना वृत्तिर्निद्रा ।

10. abhaavapratyayaalambanaa vRuttirnidraa

nidraa	Nidraa (is a)
vRuttir	modification
aalambanaa	that is associated with
pratyaya	experiencing
abhaava	the absence (of objects)

Nidraa is a modification that is associated with experiencing the absence of objects.

११. अनुभूतविषयासंप्रमोषः स्मृतिः ।

11. anubhuutavishhayaasampramoshhassmRutiH

smRutiH	Smruti modification (is)
asampramoshhas	the absence of loss, continuation (of)
anubhuuta	previously experienced
vishhaya	things (that is previous experiences)

Smruti modification is the absence of loss of previous experiences.

१२. अभ्यासवैराग्याभ्यां तन्निरोधः ।

12. abhyaasavairaagyaabhyaaM tannirodhaH

nirodhaH	The stoppage
tan	of these (modifications of the Chitta) (is to be done with)
abhyaasa	Abhyaasa (effort, as defined in 1:13 and 1:14)
vairaagya	(and) Vairaagya (detachment, as defined in 1:15 and 1:16)

The stoppage of these modifications of the chitta is to be done with Abhyaasa (effort, 1:13 and 1:14) and Vairaagya (detachment, 1:15 and 1:16).

१३. तत्र स्थितौ यत्नोऽभ्यासः ।

13. tatra sthitau yatno.abhyaasaH

abhyaasaH	Abhyaasa (is)
yatno	the effort (made)
sthitau	for (obtaining) the stability
tatra	there (in the state where modifications of the Chitta are stopped)

Abhyaasa is the effort made for obtaining the stability in the state where modifications of the Chitta are stopped.

१४. स तु दीर्घकालनैरन्तर्यसत्कारासेवितो दृढभूमिः ।

14. sa tu diirghakaalanaira.ntaryasatkaaraasevito druDhabhuumiH

tu	However
sa	it (Abhyaasa)
	(becomes)
druDhabhuumiH	firmly established
	(only when it is)
diirghakaalaH	prolonged
naira.ntaryaH	uninterrupted (and)
satkaaraasevito	respectfully practiced

However, Abhyaasa becomes firmly established only when it is prolonged, uninterrupted, and respectfully practiced.

१५. दृष्टानुश्रविकविषयवितृष्णस्य वशीकारसंज्ञा वैराग्यम् ।

15. dRushhTaanushravikavishhayavitRushhNasya vashiikaarasa.ndnyaa vairaagyaM

vairaagyaM	Vairaagya (detachment)
vashiikaarsa.ndnyaa	called Vashiikaara (is the one)
vitRushhNasya	of a person who has no desire (for)
vishhaya	things
dRushhTa	that were directly perceived (or)
anushravika	that were learned (from other sources)

Detachment called Vashiikaara, is the detachment of a person who has no desire for things directly perceived or learned from other sources.

१६. तत्परं पुरुषख्यातेर्गुणवैतृष्ण्यम् ।

16. tatparaM purushhakhyaaterguNavaitRushhNyaM

paraM	superior (to)
tat	that (Vashiikar described above, is)
vaitRushhNyaM	the detachment (from even)
guNa	the Gunas (Sattva, Rajas and Tamas)
purushhkhyaater	of a person who has realized the Self

Superior to the Vashiikar is the detachment from even the Gunas (Sattva, Rajas, and Tamas) of a person who has realized the Self. (This is called Paravairaagya.)

१७. वितर्कविचारानन्दास्मितारूपानुगमात् संप्रज्ञातः ।

17. vitarkavichaaraana.ndaasmitaaruupaanugamaat sampradnyaataH

sampradnyaataH	Sampradnyaata Samaadhi (takes place)
anugamaat	by (close) association (of the Chitta with)
vitarkaruupa	Vitarkaruupa (object of gross form)
vichaararuupa	Vichaararuupa (object of thought form)
aana.ndaruupa	Aanandaruupa (object of bliss form of Sattva Guna) (and)
asmitaaruupa	Asmitaaruupa (form of pure ego, that is ego itself. Asmitaa is defined in 2:6)

Sampradnyaata Samaadhi takes place by close association of the Chitta with objects of gross form, thought form, bliss form of Sattva Guna, and pure ego (Asmitaa, 2:6).

१८. विरामप्रत्ययाभ्यासपूर्वः संस्कारशेषोऽन्यः ।

18. viraamapratyayaabhyaasapuurvassa.nskaarasheshho.anyaH

anyaH	The other one (that is Asampradnyaata Samadhi)
abhyaasapuurvas	is result of the repetitive practice (of)
pratyaya	experiencing
viraama	stoppage (of modifications of the Chitta) (and)
sa.nksaarasheshho	the one with only impression (of existence of the Chitta)

The other one (Asampradnyaata Samadhi), is the result of a repetitive practice of experiencing stoppage of modifications of the Chitta, and has only an impression of the existence of Chitta.

१९. भवप्रत्ययो विदेहप्रकृतिलयानाम् ।

19. bhavapratyayo videhaprakRutilayaanaaM

	(The Asampradnyaata Samaadhi)
videhaanaaM	of Videhas, that is those who have been able to go beyond body consciousness (and)
prakRutilayaanaaM	of Prakrutilayas, that is those whose Chitta is merged into Prakruti or functions of nature (is)
bhavapratyayo	such that it is going to bring the experience of Bhava, that is birth-death cycle and related world, as opposite to the liberation

The Asampradnyaata Samaadhi of Videhas (who have been able to go beyond body consciousness) and of Prakrutilayas (whose Chitta is merged into Prakruti or functions of nature), again brings the experience of the world, thus not resulting in liberation.

२०. श्रद्धावीर्यस्मृतिसमाधिप्रज्ञापूर्वक इतरेषाम् ।

20. shraddhaaviiryasmRutisamaadhipradnyaapuurvaka itareshhaaM

	(The Asampradnyaata Samaadhi)
itareshhaaM	of others, that is other than Videhas and Prakrutilayas (is)
puurvaka	a result of (these:)
shraddhaa	total trust (in Kaivalya or liberation)
viirya	enthusiasm (towards reaching Kaivalya)
smRuti	remembrance (of successes during the Yoga practice)
samaadhi	Samaadhi state (3:3)
pradnyaa	Rutambharaa Pradnyaa, that is higher intellect resulting from Samaadhi (Rutambharaa Pradnyaa - 1: 48)

The Asampradnyaata Samaadhi of Yogis, other than Videhas and Prakrutilayas, is a result of these: total trust in Kaivalya (liberation), enthusiasm towards reaching Kaivalya, remembrance of successes during the Yoga practice, Samaadhi (3:3), and Rutambharaa Pradnyaa (1: 48).

२१. तीव्रसंवेगानामासन्नः ।

21. tiivrasa.nvegaanaamaasannaH

	(Samaadhi is)
aasannaH	within reach
tiivrasa.nvegaanaaM	of those whose desire and practice (for attaining it) are strong

Samaadhi is within reach of those whose desire and practice for attaining it are strong.

२२. मृदुमध्याधिमात्रत्वात्ततोऽपि विशेषः ।
22. mRudumadhyaadhimaatratvaattato.api visheshhaH

api	Also, (the Sammadhi attainment is)
tato	further
visheshhaH	graded (as being close, very close and extremely close)
mRudutvaat	due to mild intensity
madhyatvaat	medium intensity (and)
adhimaatratvaat	strong intensity
	(of desire and practice for attainment)

Also, the Samaadhi attainment is further graded as being close, very close and extremely close due to mild, medium, and strong intensity of desire and practice for attainment.

२३. ईश्वरप्रणिधानाद्वा ।
23. iishvarapraNidhaanaadvaa

	(The Asampradnyaata Samaadhi is attainable)
vaa	also
iishvarapraNidhaanad	through devotional surrender to Iishvara

The Asampradnyaata Samaadhi is also attainable through devotional surrender to Iishvara (1:24).

२४. क्लेशकर्मविपाकाशयैरपरामृष्टः पुरुषविशेष ईश्वरः ।
24. kleshakarmavipaakaashayairaparaamRushhTaH purushhavisheshha iishvaraH

iishvaraH	Iishvara (is)
visheshha	the distinguished (in a qualitative way, not physical way)
purusha	Purusha (Self)
aparaamRushhTaH	who is totally unaffected
kleshaiH	by Kleshas, that is afflictions (Avidyaa, Asmitaa, Raaga, Dvesha, Abhinivesha 2:3)
karmaiH	by Karmas, that is deeds (good, bad, and mixed, 4:7)
vipaakaiH	by Vipaakas, that is effects of Karma (Jaati - birth, Aayu - span of life, Bhoga - painful/pleasurable experiences - Chapter 2:13) (and)
aashayena	by Aashaya, that is the collection of Vaasanas (unfulfilled desires, which is same as accummulated Karma, 2:12)

Iishvara is the distinguished Purusha (Self) who is totally unaffected by Kleshas (afflictions: Avidyaa, Asmitaa, Raaga, Dvesha, Abhinivesha, 2:3), Karmas (deeds: good, bad, and mixed, 4:7), Vipaakas (effects of Karma: Jaati - birth, Aayu - span of life, Bhoga - painful/pleasurable experiences, 2:13), and by Aashaya (the collection of unfulfilled desires, 2:12).

२५. तत्र निरतिशयं सार्वज्ञ्यबीजम् ।

25. tatra niratishayaM saarvadnyyabiijaM

tatra	There (in Iishvara) (lies)
niratishayaM	the unsurpassable
saarvadnyyabiijaM	seed of omniscience

In Iishvara lies the unsurpassable seed of omniscience.

२६. स एष पूर्वेषामपि गुरुः कालेनानवच्छेदात् ।

26. sa eshha puurveshhaamapi guruH kaalenaanavachchhedaat

sa	He
eshaH	is the one who (is)
guruH	Guru (source of true knowledge)
api	even
puurveshhaam	of the ancient ones, that is the earliest sages (who realized the truth initially) (This is)
anavachchhedat	due to (his) not being limited
kaalena	by Time

He is the Guru (source of true knowledge) even of the earliest sages who realized the truth initially. This is due to his not being limited by Time.

२७. तस्य वाचकः प्रणवः ।

27. tasya vaachakaH praNavaH

vaachakaH	The verbal expression
tasya	of him (Iishvara) (is)
praNavaH	OM

The verbal expression of Iishvara is OM.

२८. तज्जपस्तदर्थभावनम् ।
28. tajjapastadarthabhaavanaM

japas	Japa, that is repetition (of)
tad	it (OM) (and)
bhaavanaM	reflection (on)
tad	its (OM)
artha	meaning ("that it represents Iishvara") (should be performed)

Japa, that is repetition of OM, and reflection on its meaning that it represents Iishvara, should be performed.

२९. ततः प्रत्यक्चेतनाधिगमोऽप्यन्तरायाभावश्च ।
29. tataH pratyakchetanaadhigamo.apya.ntaraayaabhaavashcha

apy	Also
tataH	due to that (the above practice) (two things occur:)
adhigamo	the attainment (of)
pratyakchetanaa	consciousness necessary for Self-realization
cha	and
abhaavash	absence (of)
a.ntaraya	obstacle(s in the Yoga practice)

Also, due to the above practice, two things occur: the attainment of consciousness necessary for Self-realization, and the absence of obstacles in the Yoga practice.

३०. व्याधिस्त्यानसंशयप्रमादालस्याविरतिभ्रान्तिदर्शना-
लब्धभूमिकत्वानवस्थितत्वानि चित्तविक्षेपास्तेऽन्तरायाः ।

30. vyaadhistyaanasa.nshayapramaadaalasyaaviratibhraa.ntidarshanaa-labdhabhuumikatvaanavasthitatvaani chittavikshepaaste.a.ntaraayaaH

te	Those
a.ntaraayaaH	obstacles (consist of)
chittavikshepaas	the following disturbances to the Chitta:
vyaadhi	illness
styaana	dullness in the Chitta
sa.nshaya	doubt
pramaada	nonadherance to or slippage (from the Yoga practice)
aalasya	physical and mental laziness
avirati	inability to stop (the enjoyment happening through the senses)
bhraa.ntidarshana	misconception (or overestimation of one's spiritual attainment)
alabdhabhuumikatva	not getting hold (on Yoga practice) (and)
anavasthitatva	inability to stay continuous (in Yoga practice for a prolonged time after getting a hold)

These obstacles consist of the following disturbances to the Chitta: illness, dullness in the Chitta, doubt, slippage from the Yoga practice, physical and mental laziness, inability to stop the enjoyment happening through the senses, misconception or overestimation of one's spiritual attainment, not getting hold on Yoga practice, and inability to continue Yoga practice for a prolonged time after getting a hold on it.

३१. दुःखदौर्मनस्याङ्गमेजयत्वश्वासप्रश्वासा विक्षेपसहभुवः ।

31. duHkhadaurmanasyaa.ngamejayatvashvaasaprashvaasaa vikshepasahabhuvaH

sahabhuvaH	simultaneous (to)
vikshepa	(the above) disturbances (are)
duHkha	pain
daurmanasya	dejection in mind
a.ngamejayatva	shaking of body parts (and)
shvaasaprashvaasa	uneasy breathing in and out

Simultaneous to the above disturbances are pain, dejection in mind, shaking of body parts, and uneasy breathing.

३२. तत्प्रतिषेधार्थमेकतत्त्वाभ्यासः ।

32. tatpratishhedhaarthamekatattvaabhyaasaH

pratishhedhaartham	For overcoming
tat	these (the above two)
abhyaasaH	a practice (with focus on)
eka	a single
tattva	principle
	(should be performed, if one wants a method other than
	Iishvarapranidhaana 1:23)

For overcoming the above obstacles, a practice with focus on a single principle should be performed if one wants to choose a method other than Iishvarapranidhaana (1:23).

३३. मैत्रीकरुणामुदितोपेक्षाणां सुखदुःखपुण्यापुण्यविषयाणां भावनातश्चित्तप्रसादनम् ।

33. maitriikaruNaamuditopekshaaNaaM sukhaduHkhapuNyaapuNyavishhayaaNaaM bhaavanaatashchittaprasaadanaM

prasaadanaM	The placidity (of)
chitta	the Chitta
	(essential for the progress in focus on one principle and thus towards Samaadhi)
	(is gained by)
bhaavanaatash	attitude (of)
maitrii	friendship
karuNaa	compassion
muditaa	being pleased (and)
upekshaa	avoidance
	(respectively)
vishhayaaNaaM	towards subjects (involving)
sukha	happiness
duHkha	sadness
puNya	good deeds (and)
apuNya	bad deeds

The placidity of the Chitta (which is essential for the progress in focus on one principle and thus towards Samaadhi) is gained by the attitude of friendship, compassion, being pleased, and avoidance, respectively towards subjects involving happiness, sadness, good deeds, and bad deeds.

३४. प्रच्छर्दनविधारणाभ्यां वा प्राणस्य ।

34. prachchhardanavidhaaraNaabhyaaM vaa praaNasya

vaa	Or
	(it can be gained by)
prachchhardana	intentional exhalation (and)
vidhaaraNa	intentional inhalation (or another meaning - intentional holding)
praaNasya	of air

Or it can be gained by intentional exhalation-inhalation of air, or holding air out after intentional exhalation.

३५. विषयवती वा प्रवृत्तिरुत्पन्ना मनसः स्थितिनिबन्धिनी ।

35. vishhayavatii vaa pravRuttirutpannaa manasaH sthitiniba.ndhinii

vaa	Or
pravRuttir	state (of the Chitta)
vishhayavatii	engrossed in a particular object
utpannaa	(which is) intentionally generated (even in the absence of the object) (becomes)
niba.ndhinii	responsible (for)
sthiti	steadiness
manasaH	of the mind

Or the state of the Chitta engrossed in a particular object, which is intentionally generated even in the absence of the object, becomes responsible for steadiness of the mind.

३६. विशोका वा ज्योतिष्मती ।

36. vishokaa vaa jyotishhmatii

vaa	Or
	(the same happens due to)
vishokaa	the sorrowless (state of the Chitta)
jyotishhmatii	filled with the light (of the Sattva Guna)

Or the same happens due to the sorrowless state of the Chitta filled with the light of the Sattva Guna.

३७. वीतरागविषयं वा चित्तम् ।

37. viitaraagavishhaya.nvaa chittaM

vaa	Or
	(the same happens with)
chittaM	Chitta (that has)
viitaraaga	a person whose attachments are completely attenuated (a totally detached person) (as its)
vishhaya.n	object of focus

Or the same happens with the Chitta that has a totally detached person as its object of focus.

३८. स्वप्ननिद्राज्ञानालम्बनं वा ।

38. svapnanidraadnyaanaalambanaM vaa

vaa	Or
	(the same happens when the Chitta has)
aalambanaM	support (of)
dnyaana	an experience
svapna	(during) the dream (or of)
nidraa	deep sleep

Or the same happens when the Chitta has the support of an experience during a dream or of deep sleep.

३९. यथाभिमतध्यानाद्वा ।

39. yathaabhimatadhyaanaadvaa

vaa	Or
	(to conclude, the same happens)
dhyaanad	due to uninterrupted focusing (Dhyaana, 3:2) (on)
yathaabhimata	any thing considered appropriate (by the practitioner, in order to obtain focus on a single principle)

Or to conclude, the same happens due to uninterrupted focusing (Dhyaana, 3:2) on any thing considered appropriate for obtaining focus on a single principle.

४०. परमाणुपरममहत्त्वान्तोऽस्य वशीकारः ।

40. paramaaNuparamamahattvaa.nto.asya vashiikaaraH

	(When the practice with focus on a single principle is continued)
asya	its
a.ntao	climax
	(which facilitates concentration on)
paramaaNu	minutest (object)
	(as well as)
paramamahattva	largest (object)
	(is called)
vashiikaaraH	Vashiikaar

When the practice with focus on a single principle is continued, its climax, which facilitates concentration on the minutest object as well as the largest object, is called Vashiikaar.
(This is the climax of the focus beginning with Vashiikaar Vairaagya, which is detachment from the enjoyments directly perceived or learned from external sources. 1:15)

४१. क्षीणवृत्तेरभिजातस्येव मणेर्ग्रहीतृग्रहणग्राह्येषु तत्स्थतदञ्जनतासमापत्तिः ।

41. kshiiNavRutterabhijaatasyeva maNergrahiitRugrahaNagraahyeshhu tatsthatadaJNjanataa samaapattiH

tadaJNjanataa	Absorption
kshiiNavRutter	of (the Chitta) whose modifications are extremely attenuated
tatstha	into them (which follow:)
grahiitRu	receiver of perceptions (that is, Self or Purushha)
grahaNa	means of perceptions (that is, senses (Indriya) and the Chitta)
graahya	(gross and subtle) objects of perceptions
iva	similar to that
abhijaatasya	of the Abhijaata
maNer	crystal (which is colourless on its own, but takes the colour of the surroundings)
	(is called)
samaapattiH	Samaapatti

Absorption of the Chitta whose modifications are extremely attenuated, into the receiver of perceptions (Self), the means of perceptions (senses plus Chitta), and the objects of perceptions (gross and subtle), similar to that of the Abhijaata crystal (which is colourless itself, but takes the colour of the surroundings), is called Samaapatti.

४२. तत्र शब्दार्थज्ञानविकल्पैः संकीर्णा सवितर्का समापत्तिः ।

42. tatra shabdaarthadnyaanavikalpaiH sa.nkiirNaa savitarkaa samaapattiH

tatra	There (out of the Samaapattis)
sa.nkiirNaa	that which is qualified
vikalpaiH	by Vikalpas (see 1:9 for definition of vikalpa) (of)
shabda	Shabda (word)
artha	Artha (meaning of the word)
dnyaana	Dnyaana (knowledge of the entity represented by the word) (is called)
savitarkaa samaapattiH	Savitarkaa Samaapatti

Out of the Samaapattis and that which is qualified by Vikalpas (1:9) of Shabda (word), Artha (meaning of the word), Dnyaana (knowledge of the entity represented by the word), is called Savitarkaa Samaapatti.

४३. स्मृतिपरिशुद्धौ स्वरूपशून्येवार्थमात्रनिर्भासा निर्वितर्का ।

43. smRutiparishuddhau svaruupashuunyevaarthamaatranirbhaasaa nirvitarkaa

smRutiparishuddhau	On extreme purification of the Smruti (1:11) (due to sufficient practice of Savitarkaa Samaapatti), (the Samapati)
arthamaatranirbhaasaa	which is qualified by the meaning alone (and)
iva	as if
svaruupashuunyaa	devoid of meditator's identity (not needing connection of meditator with meditation, and in which only meditated object only persists) (is called)
nirvitarkaa	Nirvitarkaa (Samapatti)

On extreme purification of the Smruti (1:11) due to sufficient practice of Savitarkaa Samaapatti, the Samaapatti qualified by the meaning alone, and as if devoid of the meditator's identify, is called Nirvitarkaa Samapatti. (It does not need connection of the meditator with meditation, and it contains only the meditated object qualified by its meaning alone.)

44. etayaiva savichaaraa nirvichaaraa cha suukshmavishhayaa vyaakhyaataaH

etayaiva	Similarly (as in the above two sutras)
savichaaraa	Savichaaraa
cha	and
nirvichaaraa	Nirvichaaraa (Samaapattis)
suukshmavishhayaa	the ones with the object of meditation being very subtle (more than that in the above two samaapattis)
vyaakhyaataaH	are described

Similarly, Savichaaraa and Nirvichaaraa Samaapattis, with the object of meditation being very subtle, are described. ('Similarly' means similar to 1:42, 1:43)

45. suukshmavishhayatvaM chaali.ngaparyavasaanaM

cha	And (this)
suukshmavishhayatvaM	becoming subtler (of the object of meditation) (is)
paryavasaanaM	such that it culminates (in)
alin.ga	Alinga (Prakruti, which produces three gunas)

And this becoming subtler of the object of meditation culminates in Alinga (Prakruti, from which the three Gunas, Sattva, Rajas, and Tamas are born).

46. taa eva sabiijaH samaadhiH

taa	These (samapattis with subtle object)
eva	very (constitute)
sabeejaH	Sabeeja (the one with a seed)
samaadhiH	Samadhi

These very Samaapattis (with subtle objects) constitute Sabeeja Samadhi, the one with a seed. (Because they still have seed made up of unfulfilled desires resulting in the birth-death cycle.)

४७. निर्विचारवैशारद्येऽध्यात्मप्रसादः ।

47. nirvichaaravaishaaradye.adhyaatmaprasaadaH

vaishaaradye	Upon reaching expertise (in)
nirvichaara	Nirvaachaaraa Samaapatti (1:44)
prasaadaH	the emergence (of)
adhyatma	true spirituality
	(occurs)

Upon reaching expertise in Nirvaacharaa Samaapatti (1:44), the emergence of true spirituality occurs.

४८. ऋतम्भरा तत्र प्रज्ञा ।

48.Rumbharaa tatra pradnyaa

tatra	There (where true spirituality has emerged, 1:47)
pradnyaa	intellectual faculty (of mind which deals with making conclusions from perceptions)
	(becomes)
Rutam	truth
bharaa	filled

Where the true spirituality has emerged (1:47), there the intellectual faculty of mind (which deals with making conclusions from perceptions) becomes truth-filled. (i.e. It understands the objects of perception in a correct and complete way.)

४९. श्रुतानुमानप्रज्ञाभ्यामन्यविषया विशेषार्थत्वात् ।

49. shrutaanumaanapradnyaabhyaamanyavishhayaa visheshhaarthatvaat

visheshharthatvaat	Due to special (subtle, complete and correct) meaning
	(Rutambharaa Pradnyaa, the truth-filled intellect, 1:48 is)
anyavishhayaa	associated with the content which is different
	(than that of)
shrutapradnyaa	the intellect used for external instruction (such as the Vedas) (and)
anumaanapradnyaa	the intellect used for making deductions

Due to subtle, complete and correct meaning, the Rutambharaa Pradnyaa (truth-filled intellect, 1:48) has a content which is different than the content of the intellects used for external instruction such as the Vedas, and for making deductions.

५०. तज्जः संस्कारोऽन्यसंस्कारप्रतिबन्धी ।

50. tajjassa.nskaaro.anyasa.nskaarapratiba.ndhii

sa.nskaaro	The impression
tajjas	resulting from that (Rutambharaa Pradnyaa, 1:48)
	(is)
pratiba.ndhii	prohibitor (of)
anya	(all) other
sa.nskaara	impression(s)

The impression resulting from the Rutambharaa Pradnyaa (1:48) is prohibitor of all other impressions.

५१. तस्यापि निरोधे सर्वनिरोधान्निर्बीजः समाधिः ।

51. tasyaapi nirodhe sarvanirodhaannirbiijassamaadhiH

sarvanirodhaan	Due to the stoppage of all (Vruttis)
nirodhe	upon stoppage
tasyaapi	of even that (single impression due to the truth filled intellect)
	(the)
nirbiijas	Nirbiija
samaadhiH	Samaadhi
	(that is the seedless Samaadhi takes place)

Due to the stoppage of all Vruttis upon stoppage of even that single impression (1:50), the Nirbiija Samaadhi, that is the seedless Samaadhi takes place.

इति श्रीपातञ्जले योगशास्त्रे समाधिनिर्देशो नाम प्रथमः पादः ।

iti shriipaataJNjale yogashaastre samaadhinirdesho naama prathamaH paadaH

iti	Thus concludes
prathamaH	the first
paadaH	Chapter
naama	named
samaadhinirdesho	Samaadhi Nirdesha
yogashaastre	in the Spiritual Science of Yoga
shriipaataJNjale	composed by the sage Patanjali (shrii - divine or spiritual, this qualifies the word 'yogashaastre')

Thus concludes the first chapter named Samaadhi Nirdeshha in the Spiritual Science of Yoga composed by the sage Patanjali.

ॐ शान्तिश्शान्तिश्शान्तिः ।

OM shaa.ntishshaa.ntishshaa.ntiH
OM. Let there be peace, peace peace.

ॐ

अथ श्रीपातञ्जलयोगदर्शनम् - साधनपादः ।
atha shriipaataJNjalayogadarshanaM saadhanapaadaH

atha	Thus follows
shrii	the divine
yogadarshanaM	treatise on the science of yoga
paataJNjala	composed by the sage Patanjali
saadhanapaadaH	Chapter Saadhanapaada (which deals with practices of Yoga)

Thus follows the divine treatise on the science of Yoga composed by the sage Patanjali. This is Chapter Saadhanapaada, which deals with practices of Yoga.

१. तपःस्वाध्यायेश्वरप्रणिधानानि क्रियायोगः ।
1. tapassvaadhyaayeshvarapraNidhaanaani kriyaayogaH

kriyaayogaH	Kriyaayoga (is a practice made up of)
tapas	Tapas (control of body-mind-speech faculty)
svaadhyaaya	Svaadhyaaya (study of spiritual scriptures from the self-realized Yogis and a regular spiritual practice such as Japa) (and)
iishvarapraNidhaana	Iishvarapranidhaana (performing all bodily and mental works with devotion to Iishwara)

Kriyaayoga is a practice made up of Tapas (control of body-mind-speech faculty), Svaadhyaaya (study of spiritual scriptures from the self-realized Yogis and a regular spiritual practice such as Japa), and Iishvarapranidhaana (performing all bodily and mental works with devotion to Iishwara) (1:24).

२. समाधिभावनार्थः क्लेशतनूकरणार्थश्च ।
2. samaadhibhaavanaarthaH kleshatanuukaraNaarthashcha

	(The Kriyaayoga is)
samaadhibhaavanaarthaH	meant for developing focus necessary for Samaadhi (1:17, 1:18, 1:46, 1:51, 3:3)
cha	and
tanuukaraNaarthash	meant for reduction (of)
klesha	Klesha(s) (described next)

The Kriyaayoga is meant for developing focus necessary for Samaadhi (1:17, 1:18, 1:46, 1:51, 3:3) and for reduction of Kleshas (described next).

३. अविद्यास्मितारागद्वेषाभिनिवेशाः क्लेशाः ।

3. avidyaasmitaaraagadveshhaabhiniveshaaH kleshaaH

kleshaaH	Kleshas (are)
avidyaa	Avidyaa
asmitaa	Asmitaa
raaga	Raaga
dvesha	Dvesha (and)
abhinivesha	Abhinivesha

Kleshas are Avidyaa, Asmitaa, Raaga, Dvesha, and Abhinivesha.

४. अविद्या क्षेत्रमुत्तरेषां प्रसुप्ततनुविच्छिन्नोदाराणाम् ।

4. avidyaa kshetramuttareshhaaM prasuptatanuvichchhinnodaaraaNaaM

avidyaa	Avidyaa (is)
kshetram	the field (for the birth as well as play of)
uttareshhaaM	the subsequent ones (subsequent Kleshas, that is Asmitaa, Raaga, Dvesha, and Abhinivesha)
	(all of which can exist either as)
prasupta	totally dormant (or)
tanu	very weak (or)
vichchhinna	ready for expression (or)
udaara	totally expressed

Avidyaa is the field for birth and play of the subsequent Kleshas (Asmitaa, Raaga, Dvesha, and Abhinivesha), all of which can exist either as totally dormant, very weak, ready for expression, or totally expressed.

५. अनित्याशुचिदुःखानात्मसु नित्यशुचिसुखात्मख्यातिरविद्या ।

5. anityaashuchiduHkhaanaatmasu nityashuchisukhaatmakhyaatiravidyaa

avidyaa	Avidyaa (is)
khyaatir	experience (of)
nitya	permanent (in)
anitya	impermanent
shuchi	clean (in)
ashuchi	unclean
sukha	pleasure (in)
duHkha	pain (and)
aatma	Self (in)
anaatma	non-Self

Avidyaa is an experience of permanent in impermanent, clean in unclean, pleasure in pain, and Self in non-Self. (This is called nature [Svaruupa] of the Avidyaa.)

६. दृग्दर्शनशक्त्योरेकात्मतेवास्मिता ।

6. dRugdarshanashaktyorekaatmatevaasmitaa

asmitaa	Asmitaa (is the experience)
	(that there is)
iva	as if
ekaatmataa	oneness (between)
dRugshakti	witnessing power, DrashhtRu (Self) (and)
darshanashakti	perceiving power, Chitta

Asmitaa is the experience that there is as if oneness between the Self and the Chitta.

७. सुखानुशयी रागः ।

7. sukhaanushayii raagaH

raagaH	Raaga (is the attachment)
anushayii	which follows
sukha	pleasurable experience(s)

Raaga is the attachment which follows pleasurable experiences.

८. दुःखानुशयी द्वेषः ।

8. duHkhaanushayii dveshhaH

dveshhaH	Dveshha (is the repulsion)
anushayii	which follows
duHkha	painful experience(s)

Dveshha is the repulsion which follows painful experiences.

९. स्वरसवाही विदुषोऽपि तन्वनुबंधोऽभिनिवेशः ।

9. svarasavaahii vidushho.api tanvanuba.ndho.abhiniveshaH

abhiniveshaH	Abhinivesha (is an)
anuba.ndho	attachment (to the)
tanu	body
svarasavaahii	which flows on its own accord
api	even
	(in the case)
vidushho	of a learned or intelligent person

Abhinivesha is an attachment to the body which flows on its own accord, even in the case of a learned or intelligent person.

१०. ते प्रतिप्रसवहेयाः सूक्ष्माः ।

10. te pratiprasavaheyaaH suukshmaaH

	(When)
te	these (the Kleshas are)
suukshmaaH	very subtle
heyaaH	(they are) removable (using)
pratiprasava	Pratiprasava (which is merging of result into its cause)

When the Kleshas are very subtle, they are removable using Pratiprasava (merging of result into its cause).

११. ध्यानहेयास्तद्वृत्तयः ।

11. dhyaanaheyaastadvRuttayaH

	(When the Kleshas have grown into)
tadvRuttayaH	their Vrutii forms (as modifications of Chitta)
	(they are)
heyaas	removable (by)
dhyaana	Dhyaana (mature stage of meditation, 3:2)

When the Kleshas have grown into their gross form (Vruttis), they are removable using Dhyaana (3:2).

१२. क्लेशमूलः कर्माशयो दृष्टादृष्टजन्मवेदनीयः ।

12. kleshamuulaH karmaashayo dRushhTaadRushhTajanmavedaniiyaH

karmaashayo	Accummulation of Karma (is)
kleshamuuulaH	which grows out of the Kleshas (and is)
vedaniiyaH	to be experienced (in)
dRushhTajanma	the seen (current) life (and)
adrushhTajanma	the unseen (future) life (lives)

Accummulation of Karma grows out of the Kleshas and is to be experienced in the current life and future lives.

१३. सति मूले तद्विपाको जात्यायुर्भोगाः ।

13. sati muule tadvipaako jaatyaayurbhogaaH

muule sati	As long as the root (made up of the Kleshas) exists (in the Chitta)
vipaako	the result (of)
tad	that (the Karmaashaya)
	(takes place in the form of)
jaaty	(particular) species
aayu	(particular) span of life (and)
bhoga	(particular) experiences

As long as the root made up of the Kleshas exists in the Chitta, the result of the Karmaashaya takes place in the form of Jaati (particular species), Aayu (particular span of life), and Bhoga (particular experiences).

१४. ते ल्हादपरितापफलाः पुण्यापुण्यहेतुत्वात् ।

14.te hlaadaparitaapaphalaaH puNyaapuNyahetutvaat

te	They (Jaati, Aayu, and Bhoga) (are)
phalaaH	with the fruits (of)
hlaada	pleasure (and)
paritaapa	pain
	(respectively)
hetutvaat	caused by
puNya	the good deeds (and)
apuNya	the bad deeds

They (Jaati, Aayu, and Bhoga) are containing the fruits of pleasure and pain, respectively caused by good and bad deeds. (This pertains to a common person, not a Vivekin described next.)

15. pariNaamataapasa.nskaaraduHkhairguNavRuttivirodhaachcha duHkhameva sàrvaM vivekinaH

vivekinaH	For a Vivekin (who has developed the faculty of discrimination between the real and the unreal)
sarvaM	everything (everything including the pleasurable Jaati, Aayu, and Bhoga) (is)
duHkham	pain
eva	only (alone) (This is due to)
parinaamadhukhkha	the pain from the change of previously pleasurable things into painful ones
taapadhukha	the pain from the troubles taken to obtain and retain pleasurable things (and)
sa.nskaaradhukha	the pain from birth-death cycles due to Sanskaaras or Karmic impressions
cha	And (this is also)
virodhaach	due to the conflict (amongst)
vrutti	the (three) Vruttis (Sattvika, Raajasika, and Taamasika) (consisting of three)
guNa	Gunas (Sattva, Rajas, Tamas)

For a Vivekin (who has developed the faculty of discrimination between the real and the unreal), everything including pleasurable Jaati, Aayu, and Bhoga is pain alone. This is due to the pain from the change of previously pleasurable things into painful ones, the pain from troubles taken to obtain and retain pleasurable things, and the pain from birth-death cycles resulting from Karmic impressions. And this is also due to the conflict amongst the three Vruttis (Sattvika, Raajasika, and Taamasika) consisting of the three Gunas (Sattva, Rajas, Tamas).

१६. हेयं दुःखमनागतम् ।

16. heyaM duHkhamanaagataM

duHkham	The pain
anaagataM	which has not yet arrived or actualized
heyaM	(is called) Heya, the one which should be removed

The pain which has not yet actualized is called Heya, the one which should be removed.

१७. द्रष्टृदृश्ययोः संयोगो हेयहेतुः ।

17. drashhTRudRushyayoH sa.nyogo heyahetuH

hetuH	The cause (of)
heya	Heya (is)
sa.nyogo	mixing (of)
drashhTRu	Drashhtru (Self) (and)
dRushya	Drushya (defined next)

The cause of Heya (2:16) is mixing of Drashhtru (Self) and Drushya (defined next).

१८. प्रकाशक्रियास्थितिशीलं भूतेन्द्रियात्मकं भोगापवर्गार्थं दृश्यम् ।

18. prakaashakriyaasthitishiilaM bhuute.ndriyaatmakaM bhogaapavargaarthaM dRushyaM

dRushyaM	Drushya (is)
a) aatmakaM	a) made up of
bhuuta	Mahaabhuutas (Aapa - water, Teja - energy, Vaayuu - wind, Aakaasha - sky and Agni - fire) (and)
i.ndriya	Indriyas (Karmendriya: faculty for activity, Dnyaanendriya: faculty for perception, and Antahkarana: faculty which receives the perceptions)
b) prakaashshiila	b) luminous (due to the Sattva Guna)
kriyaashiila	active (due to the Rajas Guna) (and)
sthitishiila	inert (due to the Tamas Guna)
c) bhogaarthaM	c) meant for worldy experiences (and)
apavargaarthaM	meant for (prompting towards) spiritual liberation

Drushya is made up of Mahaaabhuutas (earth, water, wind, sky, and fire) and Indriyas (Karmendriyas: the faculty for activity, Dnyaanendriyas: the faculty for perception, and Antahkarana: the faculty which receives the perceptions). (This is the composition of Drushya.)

Next, Drushya can be luminous due to the Sattva Guna, active due to the Rajas Guna, or inert due to the Tamas Guna. (This is the nature of Drushya.)

And Drushya is meant for worldy experiences and prompting towards liberation. (This is the purpose of Drushya.)

१९. विशेषाविशेषलिङ्गमात्रालिङ्गानि गुणपर्वाणि ।

19. visheshhaavisheshhali.ngamaatraali.ngaani guNaparvaaNi

viheshha	Vishesha
avisheshha	Avishesha
li.ngamaatra	Lingamaatra (and)
ali.nga	Alinga (are)
parvaaNi	states (of)
guNa	Gunas

Vishesha, Avishesha, Lingamaatra, and Alinga are states of Gunas. (In Drushya, five mahaabhutas, five karmendriyas, five dnyaanendriyas, and Antahkarana constitute sixteen tattvas or elements, which form the Visheshha state. The subtler form of these sixteen consists of six elements, that is five Tanmaatraas [subtle elements] and their root cause Asmitaa [pure ego]. They form the Avisheshha state. These subtler elements come out of Mahat, which is the Lingamaatra state. And, lastly, the Prakruti which does not merge into anything else is the Alinga state of Gunas.) (This is the expanse of Drushya.)

२०. द्रष्टा दृशिमात्रः शुद्धोऽपि प्रत्ययानुपश्यः ।

20. drashhTaa dRushimaatraH shuddho.api pratyayaanupashyaH

api	Even though
drashhTaa	Drashhtru (Self) (is)
dRushimaatraH	only a witness (and)
shuddho	absolutely pure
	(due to Avidyaa, 2:5, it is)
anupashyaH	participant (in)
pratyaya	the experiences (of the intellect)

Even though Drashtru (Self) is only a witness and absolutely pure, (due to Avidyaa 2:5,) it is a participant in the experiences of the intellect as its own experiences.

२१. तदर्थ एव दृश्यस्यात्मा ।

21. tadartha eva dRushyasyaatmaa

aatmaa	The core
drushyasya	of Drushya (2:18)
tadartha	is meant for that (Drashhtru, Self)
eva	only

The core of Drushya is meant only for the Drashhtru. (As given in 2:18, Drushya has the purpose of Bhoga [worldy experiences] and Apavarga [spiritual experiences]. In both of these, Drushya is meant for only Drashhtru. In other words, without the Drashhtru, Drushya has no meaning.)

२२. कृतार्थं प्रति नष्टमप्यनष्टं तदन्यसाधारणत्वात् ।

22. kRutaarthaM prati nashhTamapyanashhTaM tadanyasaadhaaraNatvaat

	(The Drushya is)
nashhTam	destroyed or absent
prati	for
kRutaarthaM	the one who has achieved the purpose of life
apy	but (it is)
anashhTaM	not destroyed
saadhaaraNatvaat	due to the common experience (of)
tad	it (the Drushya) (by)
anya	others (who have not achieved the purpose of life)

The Drushya is absent for the one who has achieved the purpose of life, but the Drushya is not destroyed for others who have not achieved the purpose of life. This is due to the common experience of it by them.

२३. स्वस्वामिशक्त्योः स्वरूपोपलब्धिहेतुः संयोगः ।

23. svasvaamishaktyoH svaruupopalabdhihetuH sa.nyogaH

	The mix (of)
sa.nyogaH	The mix (of)
svaamishakti	the owner power (Drashhtru) (and)
svashakti	the owned power (Drushya)
	(is the)
hetuH	cause (of) (or meant for)
upalabdhi	realization (of)
svaruupa	own form or true nature (of Drashhtru and Drushya)

The mix (Sanyoga, 2:17) of Drashhtru, the owner, and Drushya, the owned, is meant for the realization of the true nature of Drashhtru and Drushya.

२४. तस्य हेतुरविद्या ।

24. tasya heturavidyaa

avidyaa	Avidyaa (2:5) (is)
hetur	the cause
tasya	of it (Sanyoga)

Avidyaa (2:5) is the cause of Sanyoga.

२५. तदभावात्संयोगाभावो हानं तद्दृशेः कैवल्यम् ।

25. tadabhaavaatsa.nyogaabhaavo haanaM taddRusheH kaivalyaM

abhaavaat	Due to the absence (of)
tad	it (Avidyaa)
abhaavo	the absence (of)
sa.nyoga	Sanyoga
	(occurs)
tad	That (is)
kaivalyaM	the absolute state
dRusheH	of Drashhtru
haanaM	called Haana

Due to the absence of the Avidyaa, the absence of Sanyoga occurs. That is the absolute state of Drashhtru, called Haana.

२६. विवेकख्यातिरविप्लवा हानोपायः ।

26. vivekakhyaatiraviplavaa haanopaayaH

vivekakhyaatir	Vivekakhyaati, discrimination (between Drashhtru and Drushya)
aviplavaa	untainted (by obstacles such as doubt, confusion, etc.) (is)
upaayaH	the method (for obtatining)
haana	Haana (2:25)

The Vivekakhyaati (discrimination between Drashhtru and Drushya), untainted by obstacles such as doubt, confusion, etc., is the method for obtatining Haana (2:25).

२७. तस्य सप्तधा प्रान्तभूमिः प्रज्ञा ।

27. tasya saptadhaa praa.ntabhuumiH pradnyaa

pradnyaa	The intellect
tasya	of it (used in the untainted Vivekakhyaati) (is that)
praa.ntabhuumiH	place where (tendencies of Chitta) are completely absent (in a)
saptadhaa	sevenfold way

The intellect used in the untainted Vivekakhyaati is that place where tendencies of the Chitaa are completely absent in a sevenfold way. (The seven Chitta tendencies are Prepsaa, Jihaasaa, Chikiirshhaa, Shoka, Bhaya, and Atrupti.)

२८. योगाङ्गानुष्ठानादशुद्धिक्षये ज्ञानदीप्तिराविवेकख्यातेः ।

28. yogaa.ngaanushhThaanaadashuddhikshaye dnyaanadiiptiraavivekakhyaateH

kshaye	On removal (of)
ashuddhi	impurity
anushhThaanaad	due to the practice (of)
yoga.nga	Yoga limb(s) (2:29)
diiptir	the illumination (of)
dnyaana	knowledge
aavivekakhyaateH	(of) which culminates in the Vivekakhyaati (2:26, 2:27) (occurs)

On removal of impurity due to the practice of the Yoga Limbs (2:29), the illumination of knowledge culminating in the Vivekakhyaati (2:26, 2:27) occurs.

२९. यमनियमासनप्राणायामप्रत्याहारधारणाध्यानसमाधयोऽष्टावङ्गानि ।

29. yamaniyamaasanapraaNaayaamapratyaahaaradhaaraNaadhyaanasamaadhayo.ashhTaava.ngaani

yama	Yama
niyama	Niyama
aasana	Aasana
praaNaayaama	Praanaayaama
pratyaahaara	Pratyaahaara
dhaaraNaa	Dhaaranaa
dhyaana	Dhyaana (and)
samaadhi	Samaadhi (are)
ashhTau	the eight
a.ngaani	limbs (of Yoga)

Yama, Niyama, Aasana, Praanaayaama, Pratyaahaara, Dhaaranaa, Dhyaana, and Samaadhi are the eight limbs of Yoga.

३०. अहिंसासत्यास्तेयब्रह्मचर्यापरिग्रहाः यमाः ।

30. ahi.nsaasatyaasteyabrahmacharyaaparigrahaaH yamaaH

ahi.nsaa	Ahinsaa that is non-injury
satya	Satya that is truthfulness
asteya	Asteya that is non-stealing
brahmacharya	Brahmacharya that is obsrevance of practices for realizing the Brahman including regulating sexual passion (and)
aparigraha	Aparigraha that is non-covetousness (are)
yamaaH	Yamas

Ahinsaa (non-injury), Satya (truthfulness), Asteya (non-stealing), Brahmacharya (practices for realizing the Brahman including regulating sexual passion), and Aparigraha (non-covetousness) are Yamas.

३१. जातिदेशकालसमयानवच्छिन्नाः सार्वभौमा महाव्रतम् ।

31. jaatideshakaalasamayaanavachchhinnaaH saarvabhaumaa mahaavrataM

	(Yamas)
anavachchhinnaaH	observed without any concession (for a person's)
jaati	type of birth
desha	place
kaala	time (and)
samaya	occasion
	(that is when they are)
saarvabhaumaa	universal
	(they are collectively called)
mahaavrataM	the Mahaavrata (profound observance)

Yamas, observed without any concession for a person's type of birth, place, time and occasion, that is when they are universal, they are collectively called the Mahaavrata (profound observance).

३२. शौचसन्तोषतपःस्वाध्यायेश्वरप्रणिधानानि नियमाः ।

32. shauchasa.ntoshhatapaHsvaadhyaayeshvarapraNidhaanaani niyamaaH

shaucha	Shaucha (bodily and mental cleanliness)
sa.ntoshha	Santosha (being content with what one has to live with)
tapaH	Tapa (austerity)
svaadhyaaya	Svaadhyaaya (Japa, scriptural study, etc.)
iishvarapraNidhaana	Iishvarapranidhana (performing all activities with devotion to Iishwara) (are)
niyamaaH	Niyamas

Shaucha (bodily and mental cleanliness), Santosha (being content with what one has to live with), Tapa (austerity), Svaadhyaaya (Japa, scriptural study, etc.), Iishvarapranidhana (performing all activities with devotion to Iishwara, 2:1, 1.24) are Niyamas.

३३. वितर्कबाधने प्रतिपक्षभावनम् ।

33. vitarkabaadhane pratipakshabhaavanaM

baadhane	During disturbance
	(in the practice of Yamas and Niyamas)
	(due to)
vitarka	Vitarkas (thoughts of bad acts)
pratipakshabhaavanaM	Pratipakshabhaavan (generating opposite thoughts)
	(should be done)

During the disturbance in the practice of Yamas and Niyamas, due to Vitarkas (thoughts of bad acts), Pratipakshabhaavan (generation of opposite thoughts) should be done.

३४. वितर्का हिंसादयः कृतकारितानुमोदिता लोभक्रोधमोहपूर्वका

मृदुमध्याधिमात्रा दुःखाज्ञानानन्तफला इति प्रतिपक्षभावनम् ।

34. vitarkaa hi.nsaadayaH kRutakaaritaanumoditaa lobhakrodhamohapuurvakaa mRudumadhyaadhimaatraa duHkhaadnyaanaanantaphalaa iti pratipakshabhaavanaM

pratipakShabhaavanaM	Pratipakshabhaavana (means thinking)
iti	as follows:
vitarkaa	Vitarkas (are)
hi.nsaadayaH	Hinsaa and others (Hinsaa, Asatya, Steya, Abrahmacharya. Parigraha which are the opposites Yamas, that is Ahinsaa, satya, Asteya, Brahmacharya, Aparigraha.) (And, similarly with opposites of Niyamas.) (These could be)
kRutaaH	performed by oneself
kaaritaaH	performed through another person (or)
anumoditaaH	encouraged (when another person is performing them) (They are)
puurvakaaH	results (of)
lobha	greed
krodha	anger
moha	delusion (They could be)
mRudu	mild
madhya	medium (or)
adhimaatra	very strong (They are)
duHkhaphalaaH	bearer of fruits of pain
adnyaanaphalaaH	bearer of fruits of ignorance (and)
ana.ntaphalaaH	bearer of innumerable (other fruits)

Pratipakshabhaavana means thinking as follows:

a) Vitarkas are the oposites of Yamas and Niyamas. They include Hinsaa, Asatya, Steya, Abrahmacharya, Parigraha, Ashaucha, Asantosha, Atapas, Asvaadhyaaya, and Non-Ishvarpranidhaana.

b) These could be performed by oneself, performed through another person, or encouraged when another person is performing them.

c) They are results of greed, anger, and delusion.

d) They can be mild, medium, or very strong.

e) They are the bearer of pain, ignorance, and innumerable other fruits.

३५. अहिंसाप्रतिष्ठायां तत्संनिधौ वैरत्यागः ।

35. ahi.nsaapratishhThaayaaM tatsannidhau vairatyaagaH

ahi.nsaapratishhThaayaaM	When Ahinsaa is perfectly established (in a person)
vairatyaagaH	(an automatic) disappearance of any enmity (by others) (occurs)
sannidhau	in the presence (of)
tat	such a person

When Ahinsaa is perfectly established in a person, an automatic disappearance of any enmity by others occurs in the presence of such a person.

३६. सत्यप्रतिष्ठायां क्रियाफलाश्रयत्वम् ।

36. satyapratishhThaayaaM kriyaaphalaashrayatvaM

satyapratishhThaayaaM	When Satya is completely established
aashrayatvaM	(an automatic) receiving (of)
kriyaaphala	the fruit(s) of an activity (occurs without the actual activity preceding it)

When Satya is completely established, an automatic receiving of the fruits of an activity occurs without the actual activity preceding it.

३७. अस्तेयप्रतिष्ठायां सर्वरत्नोपस्थानम् ।

37. asteyapratishhThaayaaM sarvaratnopasthaanaM

asteyapratishhThaayaaM	When Asteya is completely established
upasthaanaM	(an automatic) gathering (of)
sarvaratna	all (the wealth indicated as) gems (occurs) (even without any desire for oneself) (or when needed for the benefit of others)

When Asteya is completely established, an automatic gathering of all the wealth occurs (indicated as gems), even without any desire for oneself, or when needed for the benefit of others.

३८. ब्रह्मचर्यप्रतिष्ठायां वीर्यलाभः ।

38. brahmacharyapratishhThaayaaM viiryalaabhaH

brahmacharyapratishhThaayaaM	When Brahmacharya is completely established,
viiryalaabhaH	a gain of great energy (that can be used for the spiritual practice and good deeds) (occurs)

When Brahmacharya is completely established, a gain of great energy that can be used for spiritual practice and good deeds occurs.

३९. अपरिग्रहस्थैर्ये जन्मकथन्तासंबोधः ।

39. aparigrahasthairye janmakatha.antaasambodhaH

aparigrahasthairye	When Aparigraha is completely established
sambodhaH	revelation (of)
katha.ntaa	etiology (of)
janma	(the past and future) birth(s)
	(occurs)

When Aparigraha is completely established, revelation of etiology of the past and future births occurs.

४०. शौचात्स्वाङ्गजुगुप्सा परैरसंसर्गः ।

40. shauchaatsvaa.ngajugupsaa parairasa.nsargaH

shauchaat	Due to (bodily) Shaucha
	(one develops)
jugupsaa	disgust (for)
svaa.nga	one's own body (and)
asa.nsargaH	an aversion for contact
parair	with/by others (with unclean bodies)

Due to bodily Shaucha, one develops disgust for one's own body, and an aversion to contact by others with unclean bodies. Alternatively, others with unclean bodies keep away from a person with established bodily Shaucha.

४१. सत्त्वशुद्धिसौमनस्यैकाग्र्येन्द्रियजयात्मदर्शनयोग्यत्वानि च ।

41. sattvashuddhisaumanasyaikaagrye.ndriyajayaatmadarshanayogyatvaani cha

	(Due to mental Shaucha)
shuddhi	prominence (of)
sattva	Sattva Guna (which is the main constituent of the Chitta)
saumanasya	peace of mind
aikaagrya	concentration
i.ndriyajaya	control over senses
cha	and
	(finally)
yogyatva	eligibility (to obtain)
aatmadarshana	Self-realization
	(occurs)

Due to mental Shaucha, prominence of Sattva Guna, peace of mind, concentration, control over the senses, and finally, eligibility to obtain Self-realization occurs.

४२. संतोषादनुत्तमसुखलाभः ।

42. sa.ntoshhaadanuttamasukhalaabhaH

sa.ntoshaad	Due to Santosha
laabhaH	gain (of)
anuttama	incomparable
sukha	joy
	(occurs)

Due to Santosha, gain of incomparable joy occurs.

४३. कायेन्द्रियसिद्धिरशुद्धिक्षयात्तपसः ।

43. kaaye.ndriyasiddhirashuddhikshayaattapasaH

tapasaH	From Tapas
kshayaat	due to removal (of)
ashuddhi	the impurities
kayaasidhhi	extraordinary abilities pertaining to body (and)
i.ndriyasiddhi	extraordinary abilities pertaining to senses
	(are gained)

From Tapas, due to removal of the impurities, Kayaasidhhi (extraordinary abilities pertaining to the body) and Indriyasiddhi (extraordinary abilities pertaining to the senses) are gained.

४४. स्वाध्यायादिष्टदेवतासंप्रयोगः ।

44. svaadhyaayaadishhTadevataasamprayogaH

svaadhyaayaad	Due to Svaadhyaaya
samprayogaH	Samprayoga (an experience of conversation with, visualization of, possesion by, etc.)
ishhTadevataa	the worshipped deity
	(occurs)

Due to Svaadhyaaya, Samprayoga, that is an experience of conversation with, visualization of and possession by the worshipped deity, etc. occurs.

४५. समाधिसिद्धिरीश्वरप्रणिधानात् ।

45. samaadhisiddhiriishvarapraNidhaanaat

iishhvarapraNidhaanaat	Due to Iishvarapranidhaana (during daily activities and during meditation)
siddhir	success (in)
samaadhi	Samaadhi
	(occurs)

Due to Iishvarapranidhaana during daily activities and during meditation (1:23, 2:1), success in Samaadhi (3:3, 1:46, 1:51) occurs.

४६. स्थिरसुखमासनम् ।
46. sthirasukhamaasanaM

aasanaM	Aasana (must be)
sthiram	steady (and)
sukham	comfortable

Aasana must be steady and comfortable.

४७. प्रयत्नशैथिल्यानन्तसमापत्तिभ्याम् ।
47. prayatnashaithilyaana.ntasamaapattibhyaaM

	(Steady and comfortable Aasana is achieved by)
prayatnashaithilya	relaxing the tendency for any activity (and)
samapatti	(performing) Samaapatti (1: 41) (on)
ana.nta	the infinite

Steady and comfortable Aasana is achieved by relaxing the tendency for any activity, and performing Samaapatti (1: 41) on the infinite.

४८. ततो द्वन्द्वानभिघातः ।
48. tato dvandvaanabhighaataH

tato	From that (success in Aasana)
anabhighaataH	absence of pain (due to)
dvandva	duality (for example, like-dislike, heat-cold, etc.) (occurs)

From success in Aasana, absence of pain due to duality (like-dislike, heat-cold, etc.) occurs.

४९. तस्मिन्सति श्वासप्रश्वासयोर्गतिविच्छेदः प्राणायामः ।
49. tasminsati shvaasaprashvaasayorgativichchhedaH praaNaayaamaH

vichchhedaH	the manipulation or control (of)
gati	flow (of)
shvaasa	inhalation (and)
prashvaasa	exhalation (to be performed)
tasminsati	after that (disappearance of duality due to the establishment of steady and comfortable Aasana) (is called)
praaNaayaamaH	Pranaayaama

The practice of manipulation of the flow of inhalation and exhalation, to be performed after the disappearance of duality, due to the establishment of steady and comfortable Aasana, is called Pranaayaama.

५०. स तु बाह्याभ्यन्तरस्तम्भवृत्तिर्देशकालसंख्याभिः परिदृष्टो दीर्घसूक्ष्मः ।

50. sa tu baahyaabhya.ntarastambhavRuttirdeshakaalasa.nkhyaabhiH paridRushhTo diirghasuukshmaH

tu	And
sa	that (Pranayama) (can be)
baahyavRuttiH	in the form of exhalation (Rechaka)
abhya.ntaravRuttir	in the form of inhalation (Puuraka) (and)
stambhavRuttir	in the form of retention outside or inside (Kumbhaka) (The Praanaayaama is)
diirgha	long (as well as)
suukshma	subtle
paridRushhTo	measured (by) (in terms of)
desha	space
kaala	time (and)
sa.nkhyaa	counting

And the Praanaayaama can be in the form of exhalation (Rechaka), in the form of inhalation (Puuraka), or in the form of external or internal retention (Kumbhaka). The Praanaayaama is long as well as subtle, in terms of space, time, and counting.

५१. बाह्याभ्यन्तरविषयाक्षेपी चतुर्थः ।

51. baahyaabhya.ntaravishhayaakshepii chaturthaH

	(There is)
chaturthaH	fourth kind (of Praanaayaama)
aakshepii	which is without any association (with)
baahya	outside (space or)
abhya.ntara	inside (space)
vishhaya	(as its) object

There is a fourth kind of Praanaayaama, which is without any association to outside or inside space as its object. (That is, it is an effortless and automatic retention in which the breath is forgotten. This is called Kevala Kumbhaka.)

५२. ततः क्षीयते प्रकाशावरणम् ।

52. tataH kshiiyate prakaashaavaraNaM

tataH	Due to that (the practice of Praanaayaama)
aavaraNaM	the covering (of Rajas and Tamas impurities) (on)
prakaasha	the luminous Sattva guNa
kshiiyate	gets removed

Due to the practice of Praanaayaama, the covering of Rajas and Tamas impurities on the luminous Sattva Guna gets removed.

५३. धारणासु च योग्यता मनसः ।

53. dhaaraNaasu cha yogyataa manasaH

cha	And
yogyataa	the eligibility
manasaH	of the mind
dhaaraNaasu	for Dhaaranaa (focussing of Chitta, 3:1)
	(occurs)

And the eligibility of the mind for Dhaaranaa (3:1) occurs.

५४. स्वविषयासंप्रयोगे चित्तस्वरूपानुकार इवेन्द्रियाणां प्रत्याहारः ।

54. svavishhayaasa.nprayoge chittasvaruupaanukaara ive.ndriyaaNaaM pratyaahaaraH

asa.nprayoge	Upon dissociation with
svavishhaya	generally intended objects of perception
indriyaaNaaM	Indriyas'
iva	as if (sort of)
svaruupaanukara	merging into the own form
chitta	(of) the Chitta
	(that is, the Chitta itself)
	(is called)
pratyaahaaraH	Pratyaahaara

Upon dissociation with their generally intended objects of perception, Indriyas' as if merging into the Chitta itself, is called Pratyaahaara.

५५. ततः परमा वश्यतेन्द्रियाणाम् ।

55.tataH paramaa vashyate.ndriyaaNaaM

tataH	From that (Pratyaahaara)
paramaa	supreme/complete
vashyatta	control
i.ndriyaaNaaM	of senses
	(is received)

From the Pratyaahaara, supreme control over the senses is received.

इति श्रीपातञ्जले योगशास्त्रे साधननिर्देशो नाम द्वितीयः पादः ।

iti shriipaataJNjale yogashaastre saadhananirdesho naama dvitiiyaH paadaH

iti	Thus concludes
dvitiiyaH	the second
paadaH	Chapter
naama	named
saadhananirdesho	Saadhananirdesha
yogashaastre	in the Spiritual Science of Yoga
shriipaataJNjale	composed by the sage Patanjali (shrii - divine or spiritual, this qualifies the word 'yogashaastre')

Thus concludes the second chapter named Saadhananirdesha in the Spiritual Science of Yoga composed by the sage Patanjali.

ॐ शान्तिश्शान्तिश्शान्तिः ।

OM shaa.ntishshaa.ntishshaa.ntiH

OM. Let there be peace, peace peace.

Student Notes

ॐ

अथ श्रीपातञ्जलयोगदर्शनम् - विभूतिपादः ।

atha shriipaataJNjalayogadarshanaM vibhuutipaadaH

atha	Thus follows
shrii	the divine
yogadarshanaM	treatise on the science of Yoga
paataJNjala	composed by the sage Patanjali
vibhuutipaadaH	Chapter Vibhuutipaada (which deals with exceptional abilities received through the practice of meditation)

Thus follows the divine treatise on the science of Yoga composed by the sage Patanjali. This is Chapter Vibhuutipaada, which deals with exceptional abilities received through the practice of meditation.

१. देशबन्धश्चित्तस्य धारणा ।

1. deshaba.ndhashchittasya dhaaraNaa

dhaaraNaa	Dhaaranaa (is)
deshba.ndhash	confinement in a particular place or object
chittasya	of the Chitta

Dhaaranaa is confinement of the Chitta in a particular place or object.

२. तत्र प्रत्ययैकतानता ध्यानम् ।

2. tatra pratyayaikataanataa dhyaanaM

dhyaanaM	Dhyaana (is)
ekataanataa	continuity (in)
pratyaya	the experience (of being)
tatra	there (in Dhaaranaa, 3:1)

Dhyaana is a continuity in the experience of being in Dhaaranaa (3:1).

३. तदेवार्थमात्रनिर्भासं स्वरूपशून्यमिव समाधिः ।

3. tadevaarthamaatranirbhaasaM svaruupashuunyamiva samaadhiH

samaadhiH	Samaadhi (is)
tadeva	the same (as Dhyaana)
	(but)
arthamaatranirbhaasaM	without the cognition (meaning) of anything other (than the object of Dhyaana)
	(and when the Chitta is)
iva	as if
svaruupashuunyam	devoid of (understanding) its own form

Samaadhi is the same as Dhyaana, but without the cognition of anything other than the object of Dhyaana, and when the Chitta is as if devoid of understanding its own form.

४. त्रयमेकत्र संयमः ।

4. trayamekatra sa.nyamaH

ekatra	the combined
trayaM	triplet (Dhaaranaa-Dhyaana-Samaadhi)
	(is called)
sa.nyamaH	Sanyama

The combined triplet, Dhaaranaa-Dhyaana-Samaadhi, is called Sanyama.

५. तज्जयात्प्रज्ञाऽलोकः ।

5. tajjayaatpradnyaa.alokaH

jayaat	From the mastery (of)
taj	that (Sanyama)
	(occurs)
aaloka	the emergence (of)
pradnyaa	(truth-filled) intellect (Rutambharaa Pradnyaa, 1:48)

From the mastery of Sanyama occurs the emergence of the truth-filled intellect (Rutambharaa Pradnyaa, 1:48).

६. तस्य भूमिषु विनियोगः ।

6. tasya bhuumishhu viniyogaH

viniyogaH	Use
tasya	of that (the Sanyama)
	(should be made)
bhuumishhu	for (mastering the) states (states reached with Sanyama performed on various more and more subtle objects)

Use of the Sanyama should be made for mastering the states (described later) where Sanyama is performed on more and more subtle objects. (In other words, Sanyama should be used for obtaining such states that are useful for spiritual liberation. Sanyama should not be used for enjoying any associated material benefits.

७. त्रयमन्तरङ्गं पूर्वेभ्यः ।

7. trayama.ntara.ngaM puurvebhyaH

trayaM	The triplet (DhaaraNaa-Dhyaana-Samaadhi)
	(forms)
a.ntara.ngaM	internal limb (of Yoga practice)
puurvebhyaH	of (for) the earlier one (Sabiija Samaadhi which is earlier to the next one, Nirbiija Samaadhi. 3:8)

The triplet, Dhaaranaa-Dhyaana-Samaadhi, forms the internal limb of Yoga practice for the earlier one, Sabiija Samaadhi. (The later one is Nirbiijja Samaadhi. 3:8) (Sabiija - 1:46, Nirbiija - 1:51)

८. तदपि बहिरङ्गं निर्बीजस्य ।

8. tadapi bahira.ngaM nirbiijasya

api	But even
tad	that
	(is only)
bahira.ngaM	an external limb (of Yoga practice)
nirbiijasya	of (for) Nirbiija Samaadhi.

But even that (Dhaaranaa - Dhyaana - Samaadhi) is only an external limb of Yoga practice for Nirbiija Samaadhi (1:51).

९. व्युत्थाननिरोधसंस्कारयोरभिभवप्रादुर्भावौ निरोधक्षणचित्तान्वयो निरोधपरिणामः ।

9. vyutthaananirodhasa.nskaarayorabhibhavapraadurbhaavau nirodhakshaNachittaanvayo nirodhapariNaamaH

nirodhapariNaamaH	Nirodha Parinaama (of the Chitta)
	(means a Parinaama that is, modification where there is)
abhibhava	disablement (of)
vyutthaanasa.nskaara	the tendency of the Chitta towards objects of enjoyment (and)
praadurbhaava	a strong emergence (of)
nirodhasa.nskaara	the tendency of the Chitta for Nirodha (staying without modifications)
	(and when there is some)
chittanvaya	continuity of the Chitta (in)
nirodhakshaNa	the instances of Nirodha

Nirodha Parinaama of the Chitta means a modifcation where there is a disablement of the tendency of the Chitta towards objects of enjoyment, and a strong emergence of the tendency of the Chitta for Nirodha (staying without modifications, 1.2), and where there is some continuity of the Chitta in the instances of Nirodha.

१०. तस्य प्रशान्तवाहिता संस्कारात् ।

10. tasya prashaa.ntavaahitaa sa.nskaaraat

prashaa.ntavaahitaa	steady flow
tasya	of that (the Nirodhaparinaama)
	(occurs)
sa.nskaaraat	due to Sanskaara (habit of staying without fluctuations, developed through a practice. 1:13)

A steady flow of the Nirodhaparinaama (3:9) occurs due to habit of staying without fluctuations, developed through Yoga practice (1:13).

११. सर्वार्थतैकाग्रतयोः क्षयोदयौ चित्तस्य समाधिपरिणामः ।

11. sarvaarthataikaagratayoH kshayodayau chittasya samaadhipariNaamaH

samaadhipariNaamaH	Samaadhi Parinaama
chittasya	of the Chitta
	(means a modifcation with)
kshaya	cessation (of)
sarvaarthataa	attraction for multiple sense objects
	(and)
udaya	rise (of)
ekaagrataa	one-pointedness

Samaadhi Parinaama of the Chitta means a modification with a cessation of attraction for multiple sense objects and the rise of one-pointedness.

१२. शान्तोदितौ तुल्यप्रत्ययौ चित्तस्यैकाग्रतापरिणामः ।

12. shaa.ntoditau tulyapratyayau chittasyaikaagrataapariNaamaH

ekaagrataapariNaamaH	Ekaagrataa Parinaama
chittasya	of the Chitta
	(means a modification with)
tulyapratyayau	equally experienced
shaa.nta	passing instance (and)
udita	rising instance

Ekaagrataa Parinaama of the Chitta means a modification with equally experienced passing and rising instances (due to very little difference between them).

१३. एतेन भूतेन्द्रियेषु धर्मलक्षणावस्थापरिणामा व्याख्याताः ।

13. etena bhuute.ndriyeshhu dharmalakshaNaavasthaapariNaamaa vyaakhyaataaH

etena	With these (using the definitions of the Parinaamas, Nirodha , Samaadhi, Ekaagrataa)
dharmapariNaama	Dharmaparinaama
lakShaNapariNaama	Lakshanaparinaama (and)
avasthaapariNaama	Avasthaaparinaama
bhuteshhu	in Mahaabhuutas (earth, water, fire, wind, and sky) (and)
i.ndriyeshhu	in Indriyas (sense faculties for seeing, hearing, tasting, smelling and touching)
vyaakhyaataaH	are explained or defined

Using the above definitions of the Nirodha, Samaadhi, and Ekaagrataa Parinaamas, the Dharma, Lakshana, and Avasthaa Parinaamas in Mahaabhutaas (earth, water, fire, wind, and sky) and in Indriyas (sense faculties for seeing, hearing, tasting, smelling and touching) are defined.

१४. शान्तोदिताव्यपदेश्यधर्मानुपाती धर्मी ।
14. shaa.ntoditaavyapadeshyadharmaanupaatii dharmii

anupaatii	The one who continues to exist (unchanged) (through)
dharma	Dharmas (properties)
	(which are either))
shaa.nta	totally subsided (or)
udita	totally emerged (or)
avyapadeshya	totally unknown (due to lack of any emergence, but going to emerge in future, currently existing in subtle form)
	(is called)
dharmii	Dharmii

The one who continues to exist unchanged through the Dharmas (properties) which are either totally quiet, totally emerged, or unknown (due lack of any emergence), is called Dharmii.

१५. क्रमान्यत्वं परिणामान्यत्वे हेतुः ।
15. kramaanyatvaM pariNaamaanyatve hetuH

anyatvaM	the change (in)
krama	the instantaneous sequence (of Parinaama)
	(is)
hetuH	the cause
anyatve	for (of) change (in)
pariNaama	Parinaama (Dharma to Lakshana to Avasthaa)

The change in the instantaneous sequence of Parinaama is the cause of change in Parinaama (Dharma to Lakshana to Avasthaa).

१६. परिणामत्रयसंयमादतीतानागतज्ञानम् ।
16. pariNaamatrayasa.nyamaadatiitaanaagatadnyaanaM

sa.nyamaad	From Sanyama (3:4)
pariNaamatraya	on the triplet of Parinaama (Dharma, Lakshana, and Avasthaa)
dnyaanam	knowledge
	(of)
atiita	past (and)
anaagata	future
	(events takes place)

From the Sanyama (3:4) on the triplet of Parinaama (Dharma, Lakshana, and Avasthaa), knowledge of past and future events takes place.

17. shabdaarthapratyayaanaamitaretaraadhyaasaat sa.nkarastatpravibhaagasa.nyamaatsarvabhuutaRutadnyaanaM

sa.nkaras	A mixture
	(occurs)
adhyaasaat	due to association(of)
shabda	word
artha	meaning of the word (and)
pratyaya	experience or understanding from the word
itaretara	which (these three) are distinct (in place, existence, time, etc.) from one another
sa.nyamaat	From the Sanyama (3:4)
	(on the)
pravibhaaga	parts (which are Shabda, Artha, and Pratyaya)
tat	of that (this mixture)
	(comes)
dnyaanam	the knowledge (of)
Ruta	the speech (of)
sarva	all
bhuuta	animals

A mixture occurs due to association of word, meaning of the word, and experience from the word, which are distinct from one another (in place, existence, time, etc.) From the Sanyama (3:4) on the parts of this mixture (word, meaning and experience of the word) comes the knowledge of the speech of all animals.

१८. संस्कारसाक्षात्करणात्पूर्वजातिज्ञानम् ।
18. sa.nskaarasaakshaatkaraNaatpuurvajaatidnyaanaM

saakshaatkaraNaat	from direct perception (of)
sa.nskaara	impressions (of past births)
	(comes)
dnyaanam	knowledge (of)
puurvajaati	previous births

From direct perception of impressions of past births (which is a result of Sanyama on them) comes the knowledge of previous births.

१९. प्रत्ययस्य परचित्तज्ञानम् ।
19.pratyayasya parachittadnyaanaM

	(Using Sanyama, from the direct perception)
pratyayasya	of the experiences (of another person)
	(comes)
dnyaanam	knowledge (of)
parachitta	another person's (that person's) Chitta

Using Sanyama, from the direct perception of the experiences of another person, comes knowledge of that person's Chitta.

२०. न च तत्सालम्बनं तस्याविषयीभूतत्वात् ।
20. na cha tatsaalambanaM tasyaavishhayiibhuutatvaat

cha	But
tat	that (knowledge)
	(is)
na	not
saalambanaM	inclusive of the cause (of the experiences directly perceived)
avishhayiibhuutatvaat	due to (the cause) not being an object of
tasya	of that (direct perception, that is related Sanyama)

But that knowledge (3:19) is not inclusive of the cause of that experience, due to the cause not being an object of that direct perception, that is of the related Sanyama.

२१. कायरूपसंयमात्तद्ग्राह्यशक्तिस्तम्भे चक्षुःप्रकाशासंयोगेऽन्तर्धानम् ।

21. kaayaruupasa.nyamaattadgraahyashaktistambhe chakshuHprakaashaasa.nyoge.antardhaanaM

sa.nyamaat	From Sanyama(on)
kaayaruupa	form of (the Yogi's own) body
stambhe	due to (i.e. causing) suspension (of)
tad	its
graahyashakti	property to be recognized (and)
asa.nyoge	due to (i.e. making) a disjoint (between)
chakshuH	the eyes (of the viewer) (and)
prakaasha	the light (from the body of the Yogi)
antardhaanaM	the disappearance (of the Yogi's body) (occurs)

From Sanyama on the form of Yogi's own body, causing suspension of its property to be recognized, and making a disjoint between the eyes of viewers and the light from the body, the disappearance of the Yogi's body occurs.

२२. सोपक्रमं निरुपक्रमं च कर्म तत्संयमादपरान्तज्ञानमरिष्टेभ्यो वा ।

22. sopakramaM nirupakramaM cha karma tatsa.nyamaadaparaa.ntadnyaanamarishhTebhyo vaa

karma	Karma (an impression in the form of unfulfilled desires) (is either)
sopakramaM	that will manifest soon
cha	or
nirupakramaM	that which will be manifest after a long time
sa.nyamaad	From Sanyama (on)
tat	them (these two types of Karma) (thereby realizing this difference between them) (comes)
dnyaanam	the knowledge (of)
aparaa.nta	death, end
vaa	Or, (the same knowledge can come)
arishhTebhyo	from (understanding the nauture of) misfortunes (a result of Sanyama)

Karma (an impression in the form of unfulfilled desires) is either that which will manifest soon or that which will be manifest after a long time. From Sanyama on these two types of Karma (and thereby realizing this difference between them,) comes the knowledge of death. Or, the same knowledge can come from understanding the nature of misfortunes (a result of Sanyama).

२३. मैत्र्यादिषु बलानि ।

23. maitryaadishhu balaani

	(From Sanyama)
maitryaadishhu	on Maitrii- etc. (Matri, KaruNaa, Muditaa, Upekshaa - mentioned in the 1:33)
	(come)
balaani	strengths
	(in them)

From Sanyama on the Maitrii-etc. (Matrii, Karunaa, Muditaa, Upekshaa - 1:33), come strengths in them.

२४. बलेषु हस्तिबलादीनि ।

24. baleshhu hastibalaadiini

	(From Sanyama on)
baleshhu	the strengths (of elephant, etc.)
	(come)
hastibalaadini	the strengths of elephant, etc

From Sanyama on the strengths of elephant-etc., come the strengths of elephant-etc.

२५. प्रवृत्त्यालोकन्यासात्सूक्ष्मव्यवहितविप्रकृष्टज्ञानम् ।

25. pravRuttyaalokanyaasaatsuukshmavyavahitaviprakRushhTadnyaanaM

nyaasat	From the casting (of)
aaloka	light
	(that is, from illumination of)
pravRutty	intentionally created states of the Chitta (Jyotishhmati, Vishokaa 1:36)
	(comes)
dnyaanaM	the knowledge (of)
suukshma	subtle
vyavahita	obstructed
	(and)
viprakRushhTa	far away
	(objects)

From the illumination of intentionally created states of the Chitta (Vishokaa, Jyotishhmatii 1:36), comes the knowledge of subtle, obstructed, and far-away objects.

२६. भुवनज्ञानं सूर्ये संयमात् ।

26. bhuvanadnyaanaM suurye sa.nyamaat

sa.nyamaat	From Sanyama
suurye	on the Sun (comes)
dnyaanaM	knowledge (of the fourteen)
bhuvana	Bhuvanas (creations)

From Sanyama on the Sun, comes knowledge of the fourteen Bhuvanas (creations).

२७. चन्द्रे ताराव्यूहज्ञानम् ।

27. cha.ndre taaraavyuuhadnyaanaM

	(From Sanyama)
chan.dre	on the Moon (comes)
dnyaanaM	knowledge (of)
taaraavyuuha	positioning of stars

From Sanyama on the Moon, comes the knowledge of the positioning of stars.

२८. ध्रुवे तद्गतिज्ञानम् ।

28. dhruve tadgatidnyaanaM

	(From Sanyama)
dhruve	on the Polar star (comes)
dnyaanaM	knowledge (of)
tad	its
gati	movement

From Sanyama on the Polar star, comes the knowledge of its movement.

२९. नाभिचक्रे कायव्यूहज्ञानम् ।

29. naabhichakre kaayavyuuhadnyaanaM

	(From Sanyama)
naabhichakre	on the Naabhichakra (naval plexus)
	(comes)
dnyaanaM	knowledge
	(of)
kaayavyuuha	the body-arrangement

From Sanyama on the Naabhichakra (naval plexus), comes the knowledge of the body-arrangement.

३०. कण्ठकूपे क्षुत्पिपासानिवृत्तिः ।

30. kaNThakuupe kshutpipaasaanivRuttiH

	(From Sanyama)
kaNThakuupe	on the Kanthakuupa (throat-well)
nivRuttiH	disappearance
	(of)
kshut	hunger
	(and)
pipaasaa	thirst
	(occurs)

From Sanyama on the throat-well, disappearance of hunger and thirst occurs.

३१. कूर्मनाड्यां स्थैर्यम् ।

31. kuurmanaaDyaaM sthairyaM

	(From Sanyama)
kuurmanaaDyaaM	on the Kuurmanaadi (near heart)
	(comes)
sthairyaM	stability (of the mind)

From Sanyama on the Kuurmanaadi, near the heart, comes the stability of mind.

३२. मूर्धज्योतिषि सिद्धदर्शनम् ।
32. muurdhajyotishhi siddhadarshanaM

	(From Sanyama)
muurdhajyotishhi	on the Muurdhajyoti (light at the Brahmarandhra, an important spot within the skull)
	(comes)
darshanaM	a vision
	(containing)
siddha	Siddhas (Self-realized Yogis)

From Sanyama on the Muurdhajyoti (light at the Brahmarandhra, an important spot within the skull), comes a vision containing Self-realized Yogis.

३३. प्रातिभाद्वा सर्वम् ।
33. praatibhaadvaa sarvaM

vaa	And
praatibhaat	from the profound intuition (obtained through Sanyama, 3:36)
	(comes)
sarvaM	all
	(knowledge)

And from the profound intuition obtained through Sanyama (3:36), comes all knowledge.

३४. हृदये चित्तसंवित् ।
34. hRudaye chittasa.nvit

	(From Sanyama)
hRudaye	on heart
	(comes)
chittasa.nvit	the knowledge of the Chitta

From Sanyama on the heart, comes the knowledge of the Chitta.

३५. सत्त्वपुरुषयोरत्यन्तासंकीर्णयोः प्रत्ययाविशेषो भोगः परार्थत्वात्स्वार्थसंयमात्पुरुषज्ञानम् ।

35. sattvapurushhayoratya.ntaasa.nkiirNayoH pratyayaavisheshho bhogaH paraarthatvaatsvaarthasa.nyamaatpurushhadnyaanaM

pratyaya	The experience
avisheshho	which is devoid of particularity (or properness of)
sattva	Sattva (that is, Antahkarana comprised of Mana, Buddhi, Ahankaara, and Chitta) (and)
purushha	Purushha (self) (which are)
atyanta	totally
asa.nkiirNa	different from each other (is called)
bhogaH	Bhoga
paraathatvaat	Because (this Bhoga, though belonging to the Chitta,) is meant for someone else (Purushha or Svaartha, the self contained)
sa.nyamaat	from Sanyama (on)
svaartha	Svaartha (comes)
dnyaanaM	knowledge (of)
purushha	Purushha

The experience devoid of particularity of the Sattva (Antahkarana = mind-intellect-ego-Chitta) and Purushha (Self), which are totally different from each other, is called Bhoga. Because Bhoga, though belonging to the Chitta, is meant for someone else, which is Svaartha (the Self-contained one), from Sanyama on Svaartha, comes the knowledge of the Purushha (Self). (That knowledge is the understanding that "I am Purushha", the witness of the Chitta.)

३६. ततः प्रातिभश्रावणवेदनादर्शास्वादवार्ता जायन्ते ।

36. tataH praatibhashraavaNavedanaadarshaasvaadavaartaa jaayante

tataH	From that Sanyama
jaayante	come, occur (the following abilities):
praatibha	Praatibha (intuitive creative intelligence)
shraavaNa	Shraavana (special hearing of sounds otherwise not heard)
vedanaa	Vedanaa (special touch of the objects otherwise not felt to touch)
aadarsha	Aadarsha (special vision of the objects otherwise invisible)
aasvaada	Aasvaada (special taste of the objects otherwise not tasted) (and)
vaartaa	Vaartaa (special smell of objects otherwise not smelled)

From that Sanyama come the following abilities: Praatibha (intuitive creative intelligence), Shraavana (special hearing of sounds otherwise not heard), Vedanaa (special touch of objects otherwise not felt to touch), Aadarsha (special vision of objects otherwise invisible), Aasvaada (special taste of objects otherwise not tasted), and Vaartaa (special smell of objects otherwise not smelled).

३७. ते समाधावुपसर्गा व्युत्थाने सिद्धयः ।

37. te samaadhaavupasargaa vyutthaane siddhayaH

	(Though)
te	They
	(act as)
siddhayaH	Siddhis (exceptional abilities)
vyutthaane	during the outgoing state (which is opposite of Samaahita state when one is concentrating for Self-realization)
	(they are)
upasargaa	obstacles
samaadhau	in (the path to) Samaadhi (1:17, 1:18, 1:46, 1:51, 3:3)

Though they act as Siddhis (exceptional abilities) during the Chitta's outgoing state, they are obstacles in the path to Samaadhi (1:17, 1:18, 1:46, 1:51, 3:3).

३८. बन्धकारणशैथिल्यात्प्रचारसंवेदनाच्च चित्तस्य परशरीरावेशः ।

38. ba.ndhakaaraNashaithilyaatprachaarasa.nvedanaachcha chittasya parashariiraaveshaH

shaithilyaat	By loosening
bandhakaaraNa	causes of bondage (Vasanaa or impressions of Karma which bind the Chitta to the body)
cha	and
sa.nvedanaach	proper understanding (of)
prachaara	flow
chittasya	of the Chitta (within body)
	(comes the ability of)
aaveshaH	entering (into)
parashariira	another person's body

By loosening the causes of bondage of the Chitta to the body (Karmic impressions), and by properly understanding the Chitta's flow within body, comes the ability of entering into another person's body.

३९. उदानजयाज्जलपङ्ककण्टकादिष्वसङ्ग उत्क्रान्तिश्च ।

39. udaanajayaajjalapa.nkakaNTakaadishhvasa.nga utkraantishcha

jayaat	From the victory (over)
udaana	Udaana (Praana responsible for quick expulsion of unwanted stuff from the body) (comes the ability of walking)
jalapa.nkaka.NTakaadishhu	over water, mud, thorns, etc.
asa.ngaH	not getting caught (in them)
cha	and
utkraantish	leaving the body at will

From the victory over Udaana (Praana responsible for quick expulsion of unwanted stuff from the body), comes the ability of walking over water, mud, thorns, etc., without getting caught in them, and of leaving the body at will.

४०. समानजयाज्ज्वलनम् ।

40. samaanajayaajjvalanaM

jayaaj	From the victory (over)
samaana	Samaana (Praana responsible for nutrition and metabolism) (comes the ability of)
jvalanaM	producing fire or intense heat (in the body, also called Prajjvalana)

From the victory over Samaana (Praana responsible for nutrition and metabolism) comes the ability of producing intense heat in the body. (It is also called Prajjvalana.)

४१. श्रोत्राकाशयोः संबन्धसंयमादिव्यं श्रोत्रम् ।

41. shrotraakaashayoH samba.ndhasa.nyamaaddivyaM shrotraM

sa.nyamaat	From Sanyama (on)
samba.ndha	the relation (between)
shrotra	the instrument of hearing (and)
aakaasha	space
shrotraM	the instrument of hearing (becomes)
divyaM	supreme

From Sanyama on the relation between the instrument of hearing and space, the instrument of hearing becomes supreme.

४२. कायाकाशयोः संबन्धसंयमाल्लघुतूलसमापत्तेश्चाकाशगमनम् ।

42. kaayaakaashayoH samba.ndhasa.nyamaal-laghutuulasamaapatteshchaakaashagamanaM

sa.nyamaal	From Sanyama (on)
samba.ndha	the relation (between)
kaayaa	body (and)
aakaasha	space
cha	and
samaapattesh	from Samaapatti (1:41 on)
laghutuula	very light cotton-like material (comes the ability of)
aakaashagamanaM	travelling through the space

From Sanyama on the relation between the body and space, and from Samaapatti (1:41) on a very light cotton-like material, comes the ability of travelling through the space.

४३. बहिरकल्पिता वृत्तिर्महाविदेहा ततः प्रकाशावरणक्षयः ।

43. bahirakalpitaa vRuttirmahaavidehaa tataH prakaashaavaraNakshayaH

vRuttir	The Vrutti, tendency of the Chitta, (that is developed to stay)
bahir	outside of (the body) (and)
akalpitaa	independent (of the body) (is called)
mahaavidehaa	Mahaavidehaa.
tataH	From it (occurs)
kshayaH	removal (of)
aavaraNa	the cover (of Rajas and Tamas Gunas) (on the)
prakaasha	the Sattva Guna

The tendency of the Chitta that is developed to stay outside of and independent of the body is called Mahaavidehaa. From it occurs the removal of the cover of Rajas and Tamas Gunas over the Sattva Guna.

44. sthuulasvaruupasuukshmaanvayaarthavatvasa.nyamaadbhuutajayaH

sa.nyamaad	From Sanyama (on the following states of objects comes)
bhuutajayaH	Bhuutajaya (mastery over the Panchamahaabhuutas that is, earth, water, wind, energy, and space)
sthuulatva	gross state
svaruupatva	form state
suukshmatva	subtle state
anvayatva	elemental or Guna state (and)
arthavatva	meaning state

From Sanyama on the following states of objects comes Bhuutajaya (mastery over earth, water, wind, energy and space): gross state, form state, subtle state, elemental (Gunas) state, and meaning state.

४५. ततोऽणिमादिप्रादुर्भावः कायसंपत्तद्धर्मानभिघातश्च ।

45. tato.aNimaadipraadurbhaavaH kaayasampattaddharmaanabhighaatashcha

tato	From that (Bhuutajaya, 3:44) (occur)
praadurbhaavaH	the emergence (of)
aNimaadi	Animaa-etc. exceptional abilities (eight Mahaasidhhis) (and)
kaayasampat	bodily wealth (described in the next sutra, 3:46)
cha	and
anabhighaatash	the indestructibility (of)
tad	those (bodily)
dharma	qualities

From the Bhuutajaya (3:44) occur the emergence of Animaa-etc. exceptional abilities (eight Mahasiddhis), bodily wealth (3:46), and the indestructibility of those bodily qualities. (The eight Mahaasiddhis are Animaa, Mahimaa, Laghimaa, Garimaa, Praapti, Prakaamya, Iishitva, and Vashitva.)

४६. रूपलावण्यबलवज्रसंहननत्वानि कायसंपत् ।

46. ruupalaavaNyabalavajrasa.nhananatvaani kaayasampat

kaayasampat	Bodily wealth (comprises of)
ruupa	attractive form
laavaNya	superior beauty
bala	strength (and)
sa.nhananatva	firmness (of)
vajra	Vajra (celestial weapon of Indra, the king of the demigods)

Bodily wealth is comprised of attractive form, superior beauty, strength, and firmness of Vajra (celestial weapon of Indra, the king of the demigods).

४७. ग्रहणस्वरूपास्मितान्वयार्थवत्वसंयमादिन्द्रियजयः ।

47. grahaNasvaruupaasmitaanvayaarthavatvasa.nyamaadi.ndriyajayaH

sa.nyamaad	From Sanyama (on the following states, comes)
i.ndriyajayaH	Indriyajaya (mastery over the sense facutlies):
grahaNatva	a state in which the senses are absorbed in perception of objects
svaruupatva	a state in which the senses are present in their own form, that is without absorption into objects
asmitaatva	a state in which the Chitta contains a vibration of the pure ego ('I am')
anvayatva	a state in which the three Gunas alone are present (and lastly)
arthavatva	a state in which the three Gunas exhibit only their purpose (Bhoga and Apavarga, 2:18)

From Sanyama on the following states, comes Indriyajaya (mastery over the senses): a state in which the senses are absorbed in perception of objects, a state in which the senses are present in their own form, without absorption into objects, a state in which the Chitta contains a vibration of the pure ego ('I am'), a state in which the three Gunas alone are present, and lastly, a state in which the three Gunas exhibit only their purpose (Bhoga and Apavarga, 2:18).

४८. ततो मनोजवित्वं विकरणभावः प्रधानजयश्च ।

48. tato manojavitvaM vikaraNabhaavaH pradhaanajayashcha

tato	From that (Indriyajaya, 3:47) (come the following exceptional abilities)
manojavitvaM	Manojavitva (travelling at the speed of mind)
vikaraNabhavaH	Vikaranabhaava (enjoyment of objects regardless of time and space, due to Indriya being unnecessary)
cha	and
pradhaanajayash	Pradhaanajaya (mastery over the Prakriti)

From the Indriyajaya (3:47) come the following exceptional abilities: Manojavitva (travelling at the speed of mind), Vikaranabhaava (enjoyment of objects regardless of time and space, due to Indriya being unnecessary), and Pradhaanajaya (mastery over the Prakruti). (Manojavittva and Vikaranabhaava pertain to an individual person, that is Vyashhti. Pradhaanajaya pertains to all, that is Samashhti.)

४९. सत्त्वपुरुषान्यताख्यातिमात्रस्य सर्वभावाधिष्ठातृत्वं सर्वज्ञातृत्वं च ।

49. sattvapurushhaanyataakhyaatimaatrasya sarvabhaavaadhishhThaatRutvaM sarvadnyaatRutvaM cha

	(And finally come the exceptional abilities called)
sarvabhaavaadhishhThaatRutvaM	Sarva Bhaava Adhishhthaatrutva (realization that "I am the base of all experiences")
cha	and
sarvadnyaatRutvaM	Sarva Dnyaatrutva (omniscience)
khyaatimaatrasya	present in the person with realization (of)
anyataa	distinction (between)
sattva	Sattva (Antahkarana consisting of Mana, Buddhi, Chitta and Ahamkaara) (and)
purushha	Purushha (Self)

And finally come the exceptional abilities called Sarva Bhaava Adhishhthaatruttva (realization that "I am the base of all experiences") and Sarva Dnyaatruttva (omniscience), which are present in a person with realization of the distinction between Sattva (Antahkarana) and Purushha (Self).

५०. तद्वैराग्यादपि दोषबीजक्षये कैवल्यम् ।

50. tadvairaagyaadapi doshhabiijakshaye kaivalyaM

vairaagyaad	With renunciation (of)
api	even
tad	that (the above two abilities)
kshaye	due to the destruction (of)
beeja	seed (of)
doshha	impurities (which are Avidyaa, Kaama, and Karma)
	(comes)
kaivalyaM	Kaivalya (spiritual liberation, absolute state of existence)

With renunciation of even the above two abilities, due to the destruction of the seed of impurities (Avidyaa, Kaama, and Karma), comes the Kaivalya (spiritual liberation).

५१. स्थान्युपनिमन्त्रणे सङ्गस्मयाकरणं पुनरनिष्टप्रसङ्गात् ।

51. sthaanyupanima.ntraNe sa.ngasmayaakaraNaM punaranishhTaprasa.ngaat

upanima.ntraNe	When invited (by)
sthaany	demigods
	(for celestial joys)
	(there should be)
akaraNam	non-performance, absence, lack (of)
sa.nga	attachment (to these joys) (and)
smaya	self- pride (in spiritual progress)
anishhTaprasa.ngaat	due to the danger
	(of falling into the worldly life)
punar	again (after reaching the above described spiritual progress)

When invited by the demigods for celestial joys, there should be an absence of attachment to these joys and lack of self-pride in spiritual progress, due to the danger of falling back into worldly life again.

५२. क्षणतत्क्रमयोः संयमाद्विवेकजं ज्ञानम् ।

52. kshaNatatkramayoH sa.nyamaadvivekajaM dnyaanaM

sa.nyamaad	From Sanyama (on)
kshaNa	the smallest measure of time, moment (and)
tat	its
krama	transition (into the next moment)
	(comes)
dnyaanaM	the knowledge
vivekajaM	qualified by discrimination (between subtler things)

From Sanyama on the time-moment and its transition into the next moment comes the knowledge qualified by discrimination between subtler things.

५३. जातिलक्षणदेशैरन्यतानवच्छेदात् तुल्ययोस्ततः प्रतिपत्तिः ।

53. jaatilakshaNadeshairanyataanavachchhedaat tulyayostataH pratipattiH

tataH	From that (knowledge described in 3:52) (comes)
pratipattiH	the experience of distinction (even)
tulyayos	between identical objects
anyataanavachchhedat	with no known differences (of)
jaati	species
lakshaNa	qualities (and)
desha	location

From such knowledge (3:52) comes the experience of distinction even between identical objects with no known differences of species, qualities, and location.

५४. तारकं सर्वविषयं सर्वथाविषयमक्रमं चेति विवेकजं ज्ञानम् ।

54. taarakaM sarvavishhayaM sarvathaavishhayamakramaM cheti vivekajaM dnyaanaM

dnyaanaM	knowledge
vivekajaM	qualified by discrimination, as described above (3:52)
iti	thus, is
taarakaM	protective (of the knower)
sarvavishhayaM	inclusive of all topics
sarvathaavishhayam	addressive of all properties (of any topic)
cha	and
akramaM	non- sequential, that is instantaneous

The knowledge qualified by discrimination (3:52) is protective of the knower, inclusive of all topics, addressive of all properties of any topic, and non-sequential, that is instantaneous.

५५. सत्त्वपुरुषयोः शुद्धिसाम्ये कैवल्यम् ।

55.sattvapurushhayoH shuddhisaamye kaivalyaM

shuddhisaamye	Due to identical purification (of)
sattva	Sattva (the primal constituent of the Chitta) (and)
puruushha	Purushha (the Self) (comes)
kaivalyaM	Kaivalya (the spiritual liberation)

Due to identical purification of Sattva (the primal constituent of the Chitta) and Purushha (Self), comes Kaivalya (spiritual liberation). (The purification of the Chitta pertains to a complete removal of the impurities of Rajas and Tamas. The purification of Purushha pertains to removal of all qualities imparted on the Self, which is intransically pure, unchangeable, formless, a mere witness, and non-participant in Karma.)

इति श्रीपातञ्जले योगशास्त्रे विभूतिनिर्देशो नाम तृतीयः पादः ।

iti shriipaataJNjale yogashaastre vibhuutinirdesho naama tRutiiyaH paadaH

iti	Thus concludes
tRutiiyaH	the third
paadaH	Chapter
naama	named
vibhuutinirdesho	Vibhuuti Nirdeshha
yogashaastre	in the Spiritual Science of Yoga
shriipaataJNjale	composed by the sage Patanjali (shrii - divine or spiritual, this qualifies the word 'yogashaastre')

Thus concludes the third chapter named Vibhuuti Nirdesha in the Spiritual Science of Yoga composed by the sage Patanjali.

ॐ शान्तिश्शान्तिश्शान्तिः ।

OM shaa.ntishshaa.ntishshaa.ntiH

OM. Let there be peace, peace peace.

Student Notes

अथ श्रीपातञ्जलयोगदर्शनम् - कैवल्यपादः ।
atha shriipaataJNjalayogadarshanaM kaivalyapaadaH

atha	Thus follows
shrii	the divine
yogadarshanaM	treatise on the science of Yoga
paataJNjala	composed by the sage Patanjali
kaivalyapaadaH	Chapter Kaivalyapaada (which deals with liberation from birth-death cycle)

Thus follows the divine treatise on the science of Yoga composed by the sage Patanjali. This is Chapter Kaivalyapaada, which deals with spiritual liberation.

१. जन्मौषधिमन्त्रतपःसमाधिजाः सिद्धयः ।
1. janmaushhadhima.ntratapassamaadhijaaH siddhayaH

siddhayaH	Siddhis (extraordinary capabilities) (are)
janmajaaH	due to particular species
aushhadhijaaH	due to medicinal herb
ma.ntrajaaH	due to Mantra (chanting of a selected phrase)
tapasjaaH	due to Tapas (austere practice) (and)
samaadhijaaH	due to Samaadhi (Chapters 1 and 3)

Siddhis (extraordinary capabilities) are due to a particular species, medicinal herbs, Mantras (chanting of a selected phrase), Tapas (austere practice), and Samaadhi (Chapters 1 and 3).

२. जात्यन्तरपरिणामः प्रकृत्यापूरात् ।
2. jaatya.ntarapariNaamaH prakRutyaapuuraat

jaatya.ntara	The species-change
pariNaamaH	modification
	(takes places)
aapuuraat	due to an automatic filling in or flooding in
	(of necessary matter by)
prakRuty	Prakruti

The species-change modification takes places due to an automatic flooding in of necessary matter by Prakruti.

३. निमित्तमप्रयोजकं प्रकृतीनां वरणभेदस्तु ततः क्षेत्रिकवत् ।

3. nimittamaprayojakaM prakRutiinaaM varaNabhedastu tataH kshetrikavat

nimittam	The incidental cause
prakRutiinaaM	for manifestations of Prakriti (Prakrutins) (is)
aprayojakaM	non-material
tu	But
tataH	from it
varaNabhedas	removal of obstacles (occurs)
kshetrikavat	like (as in the case of) a farmer

The incidental cause for manifestations of Prakriti (Prakrutins) is non-material. But from it, removal of obstacles occurs, as in the case of a farmer. (Prakruti has inherent property of flooding in. The events play a role only in removing the obstacles. Once the obstacles are removed, the flooding in takes place automatically.)

४. निर्माणचित्तान्यस्मितामात्रात् ।

4. nirmaaNachittaanyasmitaamaatraat

nirmaaNachittany	The multiple Chittas created (by a Yogi are)
asmitaamaatraat	from the (Yogi's) Asmitaa, pure ego

The multiple Chittas created by a Yogi are from the Yogi's Asmitaa, pure ego. (Yogi creates many bodies using Bhuutajaya and Indriyajaya siddhis, described in the Sutras 3:44 & 3:47, making use of the material cause of Prakruti Aapura, that is automatic flooding in. But, the Chittas for these bodies are made from the Asmitaa.)

५. प्रवृत्तिभेदे प्रयोजकं चित्तमेकमनेकेषाम् ।

5. pravRuttibhede prayojakaM chittamekamanekeshhaaM

pravRuttibhede	In the presence of different behaviors
anekeshhaam	of many (Chittas created by a Yogi)
prayojakaM	the principal
chittam	Chitta (is only)
ekam	a single one

In the presence of different behaviors of many Chittas created by a Yogi, the principal Chitta is only a single one.

६. तत्र ध्यानजमनाशयम् ।
6. tatra dhyaanajamanaashayaM

tatra	There (Out of these Chittas)
	(the principal Chitta which is)
dhyaanajam	a meditating one, (is)
anaashayaM	without any accummulation (of Karma)

Out of these Chittas, the principal Chitta which is a meditating one, is without any accummulation of Karma.

७. कर्माशुक्लाकृष्णं योगिनस्त्रिविधमितरेषाम् ।
7. karmaashuklaakRushhNaM yoginastrividhamitareshhaaM

	(The nature of Karma is)
karmaashuklaakRushhNaM	non-white non-black (neither good nor bad)
yoginas	(in the case) of a Yogi
	(whereas it is)
trividham	threefold (good, bad or mixed)
itareshhaaM	(in the case) of others

The nature of Karma is neither good nor bad in the case of a Yogi, whereas it is three-fold (good, bad, or mixed) in the case of others.

८. ततस्तद्विपाकानुगुणानामेवाभिव्यक्तिर्वासनानाम् ।
8. tatastadvipaakaanuguNaanaamevaabhivyaktirvaasanaanaaM

tatas	By that (Yogi's Karma)
abhivyaktir	the manifestation (of)
eva	only
vaasanaanaaM	Vaasanaas(unfulfilled desires)
anuguNaanaam	which are matching (with)
tad	its (Karma's)
vipaaka	effects (Jaati, Aayu, Bhoga, 2:13)
	(takes place)

By the Yogi's Karma, the manifestation of only the Vaasanaas (unfulfilled desires) which are matching with the Karma's effects (Jaati, Aayu, Bhoga, 2:13) takes place.

९. जातिदेशकालव्यवहितानामप्यानन्तर्यं स्मृतिसंस्कारयोरेकरूपत्वात् ।

9. jaatideshakaalavyavahitaanaamapyaana.ntaryaM smRutisa.nskaarayorekaruupatvaat

	(There is a)
aana.ntaryaM	link
apy	even
vyavahitaanaam	among (the manifested Vaasanaas and Sanskaaras [initial impressions responsible for the Vaasanaas]) which are separated (by)
jaati	births
desha	places (and)
kaala	times
	(This is)
ekaruupatvaat	due to the oneness (between)
sa.nskaara	initial impressions (and)
smRuti	the memory (of the previous births)

There is a link even among these manifested Vaasanaas and Sanskaaras (initial impressions responsible for the Vaasanaas,) which are separated by births, places, and times. This is due to oneness between the initial impressions and the memory of previous births.

१०. तासामनादित्वं चाशिषो नित्यत्वात् ।

10. taasaamanaaditvaM chaashishho nityatvaat

cha	And
nityatvaat	due to the everlasting nature
aashishho	of a desire to avoid the bodily death (there exists)
anaaditvaM	an everlasting continuity without any beginning
taasaam	of them (Vaasanaas)

And due to the everlasting nature of a desire to avoid bodily death, there exists an everlasting continuity without any beginning of the Vaasanaas.

११. हेतुफलाश्रयालम्बनैः संगृहीतत्वादेषामभावे तदभावः ।

11. hetuphalaashrayaalambanaiH sa.ngRuhiitatvaadeshhaamabhaave tadabhaavaH

abhaavaH	The absence (of)
tad	these (the Vaasanaas)
	(occurs)
abhaave	with the absence
eshhaam	of these (Karma, Vipaaka, Chitta, and Vishhaya)
	(This is)
sa.ngRuhiitatvaad	due to a property of collection (of Vaasanaas)
	(which is based upon)
hetu	cause (Karma or Sanskaaras)
phala	results (Vipaakas: Jaati, Aayu, Bhoga)
aashraya	residence (Chitta) (and)
aalambana	support (Vishhayas, the objects of enjoyment)

The absence of the Vaasanas occurs with the absence of Karma, Vipaaka, Chitta, and Vishhaya. This is due to a property of collection of Vaasanas which is based upon cause (Karma), results (Vipaakas: Jaati, Aayu, Bhoga), residence (Chitta), and support (Vishhayas, objects of enjoyment).

१२. अतीतानागतं स्वरूपतोऽस्त्यध्वभेदाद्धर्माणाम् ।

12. atiitaanaagataM svaruupato.astyadhvabhedaaddharmaaNaaM

atiitaanaagataM	the past-future (of Vaasanaas)
asti	exists
svaruupato	as such
adhvabhedaad	due to the property of taking different routes (of)
dharmaaNaaM	of Dharmas

(Explanation necessary to understand this Sutra - Properies of Vaasanas are called Dharmas. These are: a) Atiita Dharmas: the past ones which are pacified by exhaustion of Karma, b) Vartamaana Dharma: the current ones which have come into effect as a fruit of Karma, and c) Anaagata Dharma: the future ones due to the Karma which has not yet actualized.)

The past-future of Vaasanaas exists as such, due to the property of Dharmas of taking different routes. (In other words, even though the presently expressed Vaasanaas could be absent as given in the Sutra 4:11, the past and future Vaasanaas exist as such.)

१३. ते व्यक्तसूक्ष्मा गुणात्मानः ।

13. te vyaktasuukshmaa guNaatmaanaH

te	Those (dharmas are)
vyakta	expressed (as present Vaasanas) (or)
suukshmaa	subtle or unexpressed (as past-future Vaasanas)
	(And they are)
guNaatmaanaH	made up of Gunas (Sattva, Rajas, and Tamas)

Those dharmas are either expressed as present Vaasanas, or unexpressed as past-future Vaasanas. And they are made up of Gunas (Sattva, Rajas, and Tamas). (Therefore to remove Vaasanas, one needs to do Pratipasava of Gunas. 2:10, 4:34)

१४. परिणामैकत्वाद्वस्तुतत्त्वम् ।

14. pariNaamaikatvaadvastutattvaM

ekatvaad	Due to the oneness (of)
pariNaama	results or modifications
	(even though the Gunas are three)
vastutattvaM	the existence of (a single) object
	(takes place)

Due to the oneness of modification, even though the Gunas are three, the existence of a single object takes place. (Note: Here the word object denotes an object present in the nature. It does not pertain to the object of meditation.)

१५. वस्तुसाम्ये चित्तभेदात्तयोर्विभक्ताः पन्थाः ।

15. vastusaamye chittabhedaattayorvibhaktaaH panthaaH

	(However, even)
vastusaamye	in the singularity of the object
chittabhedaat	due the difference in Chittas (perceiving a given object)
tayor	their (of the object and Chitta modifications)
panthaaH	paths (are)
vibhaktaaH	totally different

However, even in the singularity of the object, due the difference in Chittas perceiving a given object, paths of the object and Chitta modifications are totally different. (This means that the objects in the nature and the Chittas perceiving these objects independently tread their own paths.)

१६. न चैकचित्ततन्त्रं वस्तु तदप्रमाणकं तदा किं स्यात् ।

16. na chaikachittata.ntraM vastu tadapramaaNakaM tadaa kiM syaat

cha	And
vastu	the object (is)
na	not
ekachittata.ntraM	based upon perception of one (particular) Chitta
	(If it was based upon a particular Chitta)
tadaa	then
tad	that object
syaat	would become
apramaaNakaM	imperceptible (to others when that particular Chitta is not perceiving it)
kiM	Is it not?

And the object is not based upon perception of one particular Chitta. If it was based upon a particular Chitta, then that object would become imperceptible to others when that particular Chitta is not perceiving it. Is it not? (This does not happen. Therefore, the object is independent of Chitta.)

१७. तदुपरागापेक्षित्वाच्चित्तस्य वस्तु ज्ञाताज्ञातम् ।

17. taduparaagaapekshitvaachchittasya vastu dnyaataadnyaataM

apekshitvaach	Due to dependence (of)
tad	that (perception of an object) (on)
uparaaga	getting occupied
chittasya	by the Chitta
vastu	the object (is)
dnyaata	known (or)
adnyaataM	unknown

Due to dependence of the perception of an object on getting occupied by the Chitta, the object is either known or unknown.

१८. सदा ज्ञाताश्चित्तवृत्तयस्तत्प्रभोः पुरुषस्यापरिणामित्वात् ।

18. sadaa dnyaataashchittavRuttayastatprabhoH purushhasyaapariNaamitvaat

apariNaamitvaat	Due to the immutability
purushhasya	of the Purushha
chittavRuttayas	(all) modifications of the Chitta
dnyaataash	are known
sadaa	always
prabhoH	to the owner (of) (that is, to the Purushha)
tat	that (Chitta)

Due to the immutability of the Purushha, all modifications of the Chitta are always known to the owner of it (Purushha).

१९. न तत्स्वाभासं दृश्यत्वात् ।

19. na tatsvaabhaasaM dRushyatvaat

tat	That (The Chitta)
na	is not
svaabhaasaM	self-illumining
dRushyatvaat	due to (its) being knowable

The Chitta is not self-illumining due to its being knowable.

२०. एकसमये चोभयानवधारणम् ।

20. ekasamaye chobhayaanavadhaaraNaM

cha	And
ekasamaye	at one single time
	(there is)
anavadhaaraNaM	absence of cognition (of)
ubhaya	both (Chitta as well as external object)

And at one single time, there is an absence of cognition of both the Chitta and the external object. (In other words, external objects are cognized by the Chitta, and the Chitta is cognized by the immutable Purushha.)

२१. चित्तान्तरदृश्ये बुद्धिबुद्धेरतिप्रसङ्गः स्मृतिसंकरश्च ।

21. chittaa.ntaradRushye buddhibuddheratiprasa.ngaH smRutisa.nkarashcha

	(On assumption of)
dRushye	knowability (of)
chitta.ntara	another Chitta
	(by one Chitta)
	(there will be)
atiprasa.ngaH	Atiprasanga (infinite transitivity) (between)
buddhibuddher	known Chitta and knower Chitta (because, the second shall know the first, the third shall know the second, the fourth shall know the third, etc.)
cha	and
	(there will be)
sa.nkaras	a mixture (of all)
smRuti	the memories (associated with these Chittas)

On assumption of the knowability of a Chitta by another Chitta, there will be Atiprasanga (infinite transitivity) between known Chitta and knower Chitta, because the second Chitta shall know the first Chitta, the third Chitta shall know the second Chitta, the fourth Chitta shall know the third Chitta, etc. And there will be a mixture of all the memories associated with these Chittas. (This does not occur. Therefore, there is one Purushha who is immutable and is the knower of all Chitta Vruttis.)

२२. चितेरप्रतिसंक्रमायास्तदाकारापत्तौ स्वबुद्धिसंवेदनम् ।

22. chiterapratisa.nkramaayaastadaakaaraapattau svabuddhisa.nvedanaM

tadaakaaraapattau	Due to the property of appearing to take the form (of Buddhi or Chitta)
chiter	of Chiti (Chitishakti, Purushha)
apratisa.nkramaayaas	of the one who never goes into anything else (as it is immutable, staying as it is and where it is)
svabuddhisa.nvedanaM	the knowledge of one's own Buddhi (and in turn its Vruttis, modifications) (becomes possible)

Due to the property of appearing to take the form of Buddhi by the Chiti (Purushha), who never goes into anything else (as it is immutable, staying as it is and where it is), the knowledge of one's own Buddhi, and in turn its modifications, becomes possible.

२३. द्रष्टृदृश्योपरक्तं चित्तं सर्वार्थम् ।

23. drashhTRudRushyoparaktaM chittaM sarvaarthaM

chittaM	the Chitta
uparaktaM	being associated (with) (both)
drashhtRu	Drashhtru (and)
dRushya	Drushya (2:18) (is)
sarvaarthaM	able to know everything

The Chitta, being associated with both Drashhtru and Drushya, is able to know everything. (The Chitta knows Drashtru - Self, Darshan - means of perception, and Drushya - all perceptible universe. Therefore, it can be used to know everything.) Alternatively, it facilitates all Arthas, desired achievements for a human (Dharma, Artha, Kaama, Moksha.)

२४. तदसंख्येयवासनाभिश्चित्रमपि परार्थं संहत्यकारित्वात् ।

24. tadasa.nkhyeyavaasanaabhishchitramapi paraarthaM sa.nhatyakaaritvaat

sa.nhatyakaaritvaat	Due to (its) Sanhatyakaaritva (coming together of many material items together leading to some activity. When such an activity is always meant for someone else, it is called Paraarthataa.)
tad	that (the Chitta)
api	even though
chitram	made up of
asa.nkhyeyavaasanaabhish	innumerable Vaasanas (is)
paraarthaM	meant for someone else (Drashtru)

Due to its Sanhatyakaaritva, the Chitta, even though made up of innumerable Vaasanas, is meant for someone else (Drashtru). (Sanhatyakaaritva means coming together of many material items leading to some activity. When such an activity is always meant for someone else, it is called Paraarthataa.)

२५. विशेषदर्शिन आत्मभावभावनाविनिवृत्तिः ।

25. visheshhadarshina aatmabhaavabhaavanaavinivRuttiH

visheshhadarshinaH	For the one who has realized the Self (Visheshadarshin)
vinivRuttiH	disappearance (of)
bhaavanaa	contemplation (on)
atmabhaava	the thought "I am the Self"
	(occurs)

For the one who has realized the Self (Visheshadarshin), disappearance of contemplation on the thought "I am the Self" occurs. (That is, such contemplation is no more necessary. This is because the realized Self is ever joyful, immutable, etc.)

२६. तदा विवेकनिम्नं कैवल्यप्राग्भारं चित्तम् ।

26. tadaa vivekanimnaM kaivalyapraagbhaaraM chittaM

tadaa	Then (After realization of the Self)
chittaM	the Chitta (of a Yogi is)
kaivalyapraagbhaaraM	with the heights of Kaivalya (and)
vivekanimnaM	with the planes of Viveka

After realization of Self, the Chitta of a Yogi is with the heights of Kaivalya and the planes of Viveka. (i.e. It flows from the heights of Kaivalya to planes of Viveka.)

२७. तच्छिद्रेषु प्रत्ययान्तराणि संस्कारेभ्यः ।

27. tachchhidreshhu pratyayaa.ntaraaNi sa.nskaarebhyaH

chchidreshhu	When gaps occur (in)
tach	that (the above flow) (4:26)
sa.nskaarebhyaH	due to (previous) Sanskaaras
pratyayaa.ntaraaNi	various experiences
	(occur)

When gaps occur in the above flow (4:26) due to previous Sanskaras, various experiences occur.

२८. हानमेषां क्लेशवदुक्तम् ।

28. haanameshhaaM kleshavaduktaM

haanam	The removal (of)
eshhaaM	these (Sanskaaras and experiences)
uktaM	is stated
kleshavad	similarly to that of Kleshas (previously, te pratiprasavaheyaaH suukshmaaH, dhyaanaheyaastadvRuttayaH, 2:10, 2:11)

The removal of these Sanskaaras and experiences is stated similarly to that of the Kleshas (2:10, 2:11).

२९. प्रसंख्यानेऽप्यकुसीदस्य सर्वथा विवेकख्यातेर्धर्ममेघः समाधिः ।

29. prasa.nkhyaane.apyakusiidasya sarvathaa vivekakhyaaterdharmamegha-ssamaadhiH

akusiidasya	For (a Yogi) who does not behave with 'business mentality' (Kusiidataa) (i.e. In the case of a Yogi who is disinterested)
apy	even
prasa.nkhyaane	in the Prasankhyaana (profound Self realization with exceptional knowledge-siddhis, Sarvabhaavaadhishhthaatrutva, Sarvadnyaatrutva, 3:49)
sarvathaa	in every respect, complete
vivekakhyaater	due to Vivekakhyaati (2:26)
samaadhiH	Samadhi
dharmameghas	called Dharmamegha (occurs)

In the case of a Yogi who is disinterested even in the Prasankhyaana, a profound Self-realization with exceptional knowledge-siddhis (Sarvabhaavaadhishhthaatrutva, Sarvadnyaatrutva, 3:49), due to Vivekakhyaati in every respect (2:26), a Samaadhi called Dharmamegha occurs. (Dharmamegha means a cloud of Dharma. In such Samaadhi, showers of Dharma [goodness] are constantly falling in the life of such a Yogi.)

३०. ततः क्लेशकर्मनिवृत्तिः ।

30. tataH kleshakarmanivRuttiH

tataH	Due to that (Dharmamegha Samaadhi)
nivRuttiH	(complete) removal (of)
klesha	the five Kleshas (2:3) (and)
karma	threefold Karma (4:7) (takes place)

Due to Dharmamegha Samaadhi, complete removal of the five Kleshas (2:3) and threefold Karma (4:7) takes place.

३१. तदा सर्वावरणमलापेतस्य ज्ञानस्याऽनन्त्याज्ज्ञेयमल्पम् ।

31. tadaa sarvaavaraNamalaapetasya dnyaanasyaa.ana.ntyaajdnyeyaM alpaM

tadaa	Then (when Dharmamegha samadhi and removal of Klesha-Karmas occur)
sarvaavaraNamalaapetasya	for (a Yogi) with absence of all coverings (obstacles in knowledge)
ana.ntyaaj	due to the limitlessness (of)
dnyaanasya	knowledge (there is)
alpaM	very little
dnyeyaM	(left) to be known

When Dharmamegha Samadhi and removal of Klesha-Karmas occur, for such a yogi with absence of all obstacles, due to the limitlessness of the Yogi's knowledge, there is very little left to be known.

३२. ततः कृतार्थानां परिणामक्रमसमाप्तिर्गुणानाम् ।
32. tataH kRutaarthaanaaM pariNaamakramasamaaptirguNaanaaM

tataH	From that (when very little is left to be known)
kRutaarthaanaaM	for (these Yogis) who are totally satisfied, with nothing left to achieve
samaaptir	the end (of)
pariNaamakrama	the sequence of modifications (3:15)
guNaanaaM	of the three Gunas (from Asmitaa to gross body)
	(occurs)

When very little is left to be known, for these Yogis who are totally satisfied, with nothing left to achieve, the end of the sequence of modifications of the three Gunas (from pure ego to gross body) occurs.

३३. क्षणप्रतियोगी परिणामापरान्तनिर्ग्राह्यः क्रमः ।
33. kshaNapratiyogii pariNaamaaparaa.ntanirgraahyaH kramaH

kramaH	(This) sequence (of modification) (is)
KshaNapratiyogii	correlated by moments (and)
nirgraahyaH	is noticeable (at)
aparaa.nta	the last moment (of)
pariNaama	(that) modification

This sequence of modifications is correlated by moments, and is noticeable at the last moment of that modification.

३४. पुरुषार्थशून्यानां गुणानां प्रतिप्रसवः कैवल्यं स्वरूपप्रतिष्ठा वा चितिशक्तिरिति ।
34. purushhaarthashuunyaanaaM guNaanaaM pratiprasavaH kaivalyaM svaruupapratishhThaa vaa chitishaktiriti

purushhaarthashuunyaanaaM	For (In case of) those who do not have anything left to achieve
pratiprasavaH	the re-absorption (into the Prakruti)
guNaanaaM	of Gunas
	(takes place.)
	(And, this is known as)
kaivalyaM	Kaivalya (the absolute state in which the self does not take the form of modifications)
vaa	or
svaruupapratishhthaa	Svaruupapratishhthaa (establishment in its essential form)
	(And, it is also called)
chitishaktir	Chitishakti
iti	Thus concludes (the Paatanjala Yoga Darshana)

In case of those who do not have anything left to achieve, re-absorption of Gunas into the Prakruti takes place. This is known as Kaivalya (the absolute state in which the self does not take the form of modifications), or Svaruupapratishhthaa (establishment in its essential form). And it is also called Chitishakti. This concludes the Patanjala Yoga Darshan.

इति श्रीपातञ्जले योगशास्त्रे कैवल्यनिरूपणं नाम चतुर्थः पादः ।

iti shriipaataJNjale yogashaastre kaivalyaniruupaNaM naama chaturthaH paadaH

iti	Thus concludes
chaturthaH	the fourth
paadaH	Chapter
naama	named
kaivalyaniruupaNaM	Kaivalya Niruupana
yogashaastre	in the Spiritual Science of Yoga
shriipaataJNjale	composed by the sage Patanjali (shrii - divine or spiritual, this qualifies the word 'yogashaastre')

Thus concludes the fourth chapter named Kaivalya Niruupana in the Spiritual Science of Yoga composed by the sage Patanjali.

।। समाप्तं योगदर्शनम् ।।

samaaptaM yogadarshanaM
Thus concludes the Yogadarshana.

ॐ शान्तिश्शान्तिश्शान्तिः ।

OM shaa.ntishshaa.ntishshaa.ntiH
OM. Let there be peace, peace peace.

✿

Student Notes

Appendix I
Key to Pronunciation

Code	Key
a	u in but
aa	a in father
i	i in bit
ii	ee in meet
u	u in put
uu	oo in boot
e	a in fate
ai	ai in Kaiser
o	oa in boat
au	ow in now
aM	mm in Umm!
a.n	a.n is for Anusvaar (dot over Sanskrit letter). un in bounce or in pronounce
aH	Uh!
.a	prolongs the previous letter, for example o.a is like ow in show
k	k in skin
kh	kh in brick-head
g	g in get
gh	gh in dog-house
ch	ch in chin
chh	chh in church-hat, ch-h in march-hare
j	j in major
jh	ge-h in sledge-hammer, ge-h in page-her
JN	nch in bench, nge in change

Code	Key
T	t in stick
Th	t-h in fat-head and in boat-house
D	d in dig
Dh	d-h in head-hair, dh in adhere
N	n in band
t	t in restaurant and travaille (French)
th	th in bath, faith, and thank
d	th in then
dh	th-h in with-hold
n	n in net
p	p in spin
ph	p-h in sharp-hit
b	b in big
bh	b-H in Bob-Harry
m	m in met
y	y in yet
r	r in rat
l	l in let
v	w in wet
sh	sh in shin
shh	sh in shin with tongue moved in
s	s in sin
h	h in hat
ksh	k-sh in back-shot
tr	tra in mantra

अथ श्रीपातञ्जलयोगदर्शनम् - समाधिपादः ।

atha shriipaataJNjalayogadarshanaM samaadhipaadaH

१.अथ योगानुशासनम् ।

1. atha yogaanushaasanaM

२.योगश्चित्तवृत्तिनिरोधः ।

2. yogashchittavRuttinirodhaH

३. तदा द्रष्टुःस्वरूपेऽवस्थानम् ।

3. tadaa drashhTussvaruupe.avasthaanaM

४. वृत्तिसारूप्यमितरत्र ।

4. vRuttisaaruupyamitaratra

५. वृत्तयः पञ्चतय्यः क्लिष्टाऽक्लिष्टाः ।

5. vRuttayaH paJNchatayyaH klishhTaa.aklishhTaaH

६. प्रमाणविपर्ययविकल्पनिद्रास्मृतयः ।

6. pramaaNaviparyayavikalpanidraasmRutayaH

७. प्रत्यक्षानुमानागमाः प्रमाणानि ।

7. pratyakshaanumaanaagamaaH pramaaNaani

८. विपर्ययो मिथ्याज्ञानमतद्रूपप्रतिष्ठम् ।

8. viparyayo mithyaadnyaanamatadruupapratishhThaM

९.शब्दज्ञानानुपाती वस्तुशून्यो विकल्पः ।

9. shabdadnyaanaanupaatii vastushuunyo vikalpaH

१०.अभावप्रत्ययालम्बना वृत्तिनिद्रा ।

10. abhaavapratyayaalambanaa vRuttirnidraa

११. अनुभूतविषयासंप्रमोषः स्मृतिः ।

11. anubhuutavishhayaasampramoshhassmRutiH

१२. अभ्यासवैराग्याभ्यां तन्निरोधः ।

12. abhyaasavairaagyaabhyaaM tannirodhaH

१३. तत्र स्थितौ यत्नोऽभ्यासः ।

13. tatra sthitau yatno.abhyaasaH

१४. स तु दीर्घकालनैरन्तर्यसत्कारासेवितो दृढभूमिः ।

14. sa tu diirghakaalanaira.ntaryasatkaaraasevito druDhabhuumiH

१५. दृष्टानुश्रविकविषयवितृष्णस्य वशीकारसंज्ञा वैराग्यम् ।

15. dRushhTaanushravikavishhayavitRushhNasya vashiikaarasa.ndnyaa vairaagyaM

१६. तत्परं पुरुषख्यातेर्गुणवैतृष्ण्यम् ।

16. tatparaM purushhakhyaaterguNavaitRushhNyaM

१७. वितर्कविचारानन्दास्मितारूपानुगमात् संप्रज्ञातः ।

17. vitarkavichaaraana.ndaasmitaaruupaanugamaat sampradnyaataH

१८. विरामप्रत्ययाभ्यासपूर्वः संस्कारशेषोऽन्यः।

18. viraamapratyayaabhyaasapuurvassa.nskaarasheshho.anyaH

१९. भवप्रत्ययो विदेहप्रकृतिलयानाम् ।

19. bhavapratyayo videhaprakRutilayaanaaM

२०. श्रद्धावीर्यस्मृतिसमाधिप्रज्ञापूर्वक इतरेषाम् ।

20. shraddhaaviiryasmRutisamaadhipradnyaapuurvaka itareshhaaM

२१. तीव्रसंवेगानामासन्नः ।

21. tiivrasa.nvegaanaamaasannaH

२२. मृदुमध्याधिमात्रत्वात्ततोऽपि विशेषः ।

22. mRudumadhyaadhimaatratvaattato.api visheshhaH

२३. ईश्वरप्रणिधानाद्वा ।

23. iishvarapraNidhaanaadvaa

२४. क्लेशकर्मविपाकाशयैरपरामृष्टः पुरुषविशेष ईश्वरः ।

24. kleshakarmavipaakaashayairaparaamRushhTaH purushhavisheshha iishvaraH

२५. तत्र निरतिशयं सार्वज्ञ्यबीजम् ।

25. tatra niratishayaM saarvadnyyabiijaM

२६. स एष पूर्वेषामपि गुरुः कालेनानवच्छेदात् ।

26. sa eshha puurveshhaamapi guruH kaalenaanavachchhedaat

२७. तस्य वाचकः प्रणवः ।

27. tasya vaachakaH praNavaH

२८. तज्जपस्तदर्थभावनम् ।

28. tajjapastadarthabhaavanaM

२९. ततः प्रत्यक्चेतनाधिगमोऽप्यन्तरायाभावश्च ।

29. tataH pratyakchetanaadhigamo.apya.ntaraayaabhaavashcha

३०. व्याधिस्त्यानसंशयप्रमादालस्याविरतिभ्रान्तिदर्शना-लब्धभूमिकत्वानवस्थितत्वानि चित्तविक्षेपास्तेऽन्तरायाः ।

30. vyaadhistyaanasa.nshayapramaadaalasyaaviratibhraa.ntidarshanaa-labdhabhuumikatvaanavasthitatvaani chittavikshepaaste.a.ntaraayaaH

३१. दुःखदौर्मनस्याङ्गमेजयत्वश्वासप्रश्वासा विक्षेपसहभुवः ।

31. duHkhadaurmanasyaa.ngamejayatvashvaasaprashvaasaa vikshepasahabhuvaH

३२. तत्प्रतिषेधार्थमेकतत्त्वाभ्यासः ।

32. tatpratishhedhaarthamekatattvaabhyaasaH

३३. मैत्रीकरुणामुदितोपेक्षाणां सुखदुःखपुण्यापुण्यविषयाणां भावनातश्चित्तप्रसादनम् ।

33. maitriikaruNaamuditopekshaaNaaM sukhaduHkhapuNyaapuNyavishhayaaNaaM bhaavanaatashchittaprasaadanaM

३४. प्रच्छर्दनविधारणाभ्यां वा प्राणस्य ।

34. prachchhardanavidhaaraNaabhyaaM vaa praaNasya

३५. विषयवती वा प्रवृत्तिरुत्पन्ना मनसः स्थितिनिबन्धिनी ।

35. vishhayavatii vaa pravRuttirutpannaa manasaH sthitiniba.ndhinii

३६. विशोका वा ज्योतिष्मती ।

36. vishokaa vaa jyotishhmatii

३७. वीतरागविषयं वा चित्तम् ।

37. viitaraagavishhaya.nvaa chittaM

३८. स्वप्ननिद्राज्ञानालम्बनं वा ।

38. svapnanidraadnyaanaalambanaM vaa

३९. यथाभिमतध्यानाद्वा ।

39. yathaabhimatadhyaanaadvaa

४०. परमाणुपरममहत्त्वान्तोऽस्य वशीकारः ।

40. paramaaNuparamamahattvaa.nto.asya vashiikaaraH

४१. क्षीणवृत्तेरभिजातस्येव मणेर्ग्रहीतृग्रहणग्राह्येषु तत्स्थतदञ्जनतासमापत्तिः ।

41. kshiiNavRutterabhijaatasyeva maNergrahiitRugrahaNagraahyeshhu tatsthatadaJNjanataa samaapattiH

४२. तत्र शब्दार्थज्ञानविकल्पैः संकीर्णा सवितर्का समापत्तिः ।

42. tatra shabdaarthadnyaanavikalpaiH sa.nkiirNaa savitarkaa samaapattiH

४३. स्मृतिपरिशुद्धौ स्वरूपशून्येवार्थमात्रनिर्भासा निर्वितर्का ।

43. smRutiparishuddhau svaruupashuunyevaarthamaatranirbhaasaa nirvitarkaa

४४. एतयैव सविचारा निर्विचारा च सूक्ष्मविषया व्याख्याताः ।

44. etayaiva savichaaraa nirvichaaraa cha suukshmavishhayaa vyaakhyaataaH

४५. सूक्ष्मविषयत्वं चालिङ्गपर्यवसानम् ।

45. suukshmavishhayatvaM chaali.ngaparyavasaanaM

४६. ता एव सबीजः समाधिः ।

46. taa eva sabiijaH samaadhiH

४७. निर्विचारवैशारद्येऽध्यात्मप्रसादः ।

47. nirvichaaravaishaaradye.adhyaatmaprasaadaH

४८. ऋतम्भरा तत्र प्रज्ञा ।

48.Rumbharaa tatra pradnyaa

४९. श्रुतानुमानप्रज्ञाभ्यामन्यविषया विशेषार्थत्वात् ।

49. shrutaanumaanapradnyaabhyaamanyavishhayaa visheshhaarthatvaat

५०. तज्जः संस्कारोऽन्यसंस्कारप्रतिबन्धी ।

50. tajjassa.nskaaro.anyasa.nskaarapratiba.ndhii

५१. तस्यापि निरोधे सर्वनिरोधान्निर्बीजः समाधिः ।

51. tasyaapi nirodhe sarvanirodhaannirbiijassamaadhiH

इति श्रीपातञ्जले योगशास्त्रे समाधिनिर्देशो नाम प्रथमः पादः ।

iti shriipaataJNjale yogashaastre samaadhinirdesho naama prathamaH paadaH

ॐ शान्तिश्शान्तिश्शान्तिः ।

OM shaa.ntishshaa.ntishshaa.ntiH

अथ श्रीपातञ्जलयोगदर्शनम् - साधनपादः ।

atha shriipaataJNjalayogadarshanaM saadhanapaadaH

१. तपःस्वाध्यायेश्वरप्रणिधानानि क्रियायोगः ।

1. tapassvaadhyaayeshvarapraNidhaanaani kriyaayogaH

२. समाधिभावनार्थः क्लेशतनूकरणार्थश्च ।

2. samaadhibhaavanaarthaH kleshatanuukaraNaarthashcha

३. अविद्यास्मितारागद्वेषाभिनिवेशाः क्लेशाः ।

3. avidyaasmitaaraagadveshhaabhiniveshaaH kleshaaH

४. अविद्या क्षेत्रमुत्तरेषां प्रसुप्ततनुविच्छिन्नोदाराणाम् ।

4. avidyaa kshetramuttareshhaaM prasuptatanuvichchhinnodaaraaNaaM

५. अनित्याशुचिदुःखानात्मसु नित्यशुचिसुखात्मख्यातिरविद्या ।

5. anityaashuchiduHkhaanaatmasu nityashuchisukhaatmakhyaatiravidyaa

६. दृग्दर्शनशक्त्योरेकात्मतेवास्मिता ।

6. dRugdarshanashaktyorekaatmatevaasmitaa

७. सुखानुशयी रागः ।

7. sukhaanushayii raagaH

८. दुःखानुशयी द्वेषः ।

8. duHkhaanushayii dveshhaH

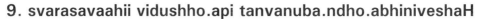

९. स्वरसवाही विदुषोऽपि तन्वनुबंधोऽभिनिवेशः ।

9. svarasavaahii vidushho.api tanvanuba.ndho.abhiniveshaH

१०. ते प्रतिप्रसवहेयाः सूक्ष्माः ।

10. te pratiprasavaheyaaH suukshmaaH

११. ध्यानहेयास्तद्वृत्तयः ।

11. dhyaanaheyaastadvRuttayaH

१२. क्लेशमूलः कर्माशयो दृष्टादृष्टजन्मवेदनीयः ।

12. kleshamuulaH karmaashayo dRushhTaadRushhTajanmavedaniiyaH

१३. सति मूले तद्विपाको जात्यायुर्भोगाः ।

13. sati muule tadvipaako jaatyaayurbhogaaH

१४. ते ह्लादपरितापफलाः पुण्यापुण्यहेतुत्वात् ।

14.te hlaadaparitaapaphalaaH puNyaapuNyahetutvaat

१५. परिणामतापसंस्कारदुःखैर्गुणवृत्तिविरोधाच्च दुःखमेव सर्व विवेकिनः ।

15. pariNaamataapasa.nskaaraduHkhairguNavRuttivirodhaachcha duHkhameva
sarvaM vivekinaH

१६. हेयं दुःखमनागतम् ।

16. heyaM duHkhamanaagataM

१७. द्रष्टृदृश्ययोः संयोगो हेयहेतुः ।

17. drashhTRudRushyayoH sa.nyogo heyahetuH

१८. प्रकाशक्रियास्थितिशीलं भूतेन्द्रियात्मकं भोगापवर्गार्थं दृश्यम् ।

18. prakaashakriyaasthitishiilaM bhuute.ndriyaatmakaM bhogaapavargaarthaM
dRushyaM

१९. विशेषाविशेषलिङ्गमात्रालिङ्गानि गुणपर्वाणि ।

19. visheshhaavisheshhali.ngamaatraali.ngaani guNaparvaaNi

२०. द्रष्टा दृशिमात्रः शुद्धोऽपि प्रत्ययानुपश्यः ।

20. drashhTaa dRushimaatraH shuddho.api pratyayaanupashyaH

२१. तदर्थ एव दृश्यस्यात्मा ।

21. tadartha eva dRushyasyaatmaa

२२. कृतार्थं प्रति नष्टमप्यनष्टं तदन्यसाधारणत्वात् ।

22. kRutaarthaM prati nashhTamapyanashhTaM tadanyasaadhaaraNatvaat

२३. स्वस्वामिशक्त्योः स्वरूपोपलब्धिहेतुः संयोगः ।

23. svasvaamishaktyoH svaruupopalabdhihetuH sa.nyogaH

२४. तस्य हेतुरविद्या ।

24. tasya heturavidyaa

२५. तदभावात्संयोगाभावो हानं तद्दृशेः कैवल्यम् ।

25. tadabhaavaatsa.nyogaabhaavo haanaM taddRusheH kaivalyaM

२६. विवेकख्यातिरविप्लवा हानोपायः ।

26. vivekakhyaatiraviplavaa haanopaayaH

२७. तस्य सप्तधा प्रान्तभूमिः प्रज्ञा ।

27. tasya saptadhaa praa.ntabhuumiH pradnyaa

२८. योगाङ्गानुष्ठानादशुद्धिक्षये ज्ञानदीसिराविवेकख्यातेः ।

28. yogaa.ngaanushhThaanaadashuddhikshaye dnyaanadiiptiraavivekakhyaateH

२९. यमनियमासनप्राणायामप्रत्याहारधारणाध्यानसमाधयोऽष्टावङ्गानि

29.yamaniyamaasanapraaNaayaamapratyaahaaradhaaraNaadhyaanasamaadhayo.as-hhTaava.ngaani

३०. अहिंसासत्यास्तेयब्रह्मचर्यापरिग्रहाः यमाः ।

30. ahi.nsaasatyaasteyabrahmacharyaaparigrahaaH yamaaH

३१. जातिदेशकालसमयानवच्छिन्नाः सार्वभौमा महाव्रतम् ।

31. jaatideshakaalasamayaanavachchhinnaaH saarvabhaumaa mahaavrataM

३२. शौचसन्तोषतपःस्वाध्यायेश्वरप्रणिधानानि नियमाः ।

32. shauchasa.ntoshhatapaHsvaadhyaayeshvarapraNidhaanaani niyamaaH

३३. वितर्कबाधने प्रतिपक्षभावनम् ।

33. vitarkabaadhane pratipakshabhaavanaM

३४. वितर्का हिंसादयः कृतकारितानुमोदिता लोभक्रोधमोहपूर्वका मृदुमध्याधिमात्रा दुःखाज्ञानानन्तफला इति प्रतिपक्षभावनम् ।

34. vitarkaa hi.nsaadayaH kRutakaaritaanumoditaa lobhakrodhamohapuurvakaa mRudumadhyaadhimaatraa duHkhaadnyaanaanantaphalaa iti pratipakshabhaavanaM

३५. अहिंसाप्रतिष्ठायां तत्संनिधौ वैरत्यागः ।

35. ahi.nsaapratishhThaayaaM tatsannidhau vairatyaagaH

३६. सत्यप्रतिष्ठायां क्रियाफलाश्रयत्वम् ।

36. satyapratishhThaayaaM kriyaaphalaashrayatvaM

३७. अस्तेयप्रतिष्ठायां सर्वरत्नोपस्थानम् ।

37. asteyapratishhThaayaaM sarvaratnopasthaanaM

३८. ब्रह्मचर्यप्रतिष्ठायां वीर्यलाभः ।

38. brahmacharyapratishhThaayaaM viiryalaabhaH

३९. अपरिग्रहस्थैर्ये जन्मकथन्तासंबोधः ।

39. aparigrahasthairye janmakatha.antaasambodhaH

४०. शौचात्स्वाङ्गजुगुप्सा परैरसंसर्गः ।

40. shauchaatsvaa.ngajugupsaa parairasa.nsargaH

४१. सत्त्वशुद्धिसौमनस्यैकाग्र्येन्द्रियजयात्मदर्शनयोग्यत्वानि च ।

41. sattvashuddhisaumanasyaikaagrye.ndriyajayaatmadarshanayogyatvaani cha

४२. संतोषादनुत्तमसुखलाभः ।

42. sa.ntoshhaadanuttamasukhalaabhaH

४३. कायेन्द्रियसिद्धिरशुद्धिक्षयात्तपसः ।

43. kaaye.ndriyasiddhirashuddhikshayaattapasaH

४४. स्वाध्यायादिष्टदेवतासंप्रयोगः ।

44. svaadhyaayaadishhTadevataasamprayogaH

४५. समाधिसिद्धिरीश्वरप्रणिधानात् ।

45. samaadhisiddhiriishvarapraNidhaanaat

४६. स्थिरसुखमासनम् ।

46. sthirasukhamaasanaM

४७. प्रयत्नशैथिल्यानन्तसमापत्तिभ्याम् ।

47. prayatnashaithilyaana.ntasamaapattibhyaaM

४८. ततो द्वन्द्वानभिघातः ।

48. tato dvandvaanabhighaataH

४९. तस्मिन्सति श्वासप्रश्वासयोर्गतिविच्छेदः प्राणायामः ।

49. tasminsati shvaasaprashvaasayorgativichchhedaH praaNaayaamaH

५०. स तु बाह्याभ्यन्तरस्तम्भवृत्तिर्देशकालसंख्याभिः परिदृष्टो दीर्घसूक्ष्मः ।

50. sa tu baahyaabhya.ntarastambhavRuttirdeshakaalasa.nkhyaabhiH paridRushhTo diirghasuukshmaH

५१. बाह्याभ्यन्तरविषयाक्षेपी चतुर्थः ।

51. baahyaabhya.ntaravishhayaakshepii chaturthaH

५२. ततः क्षीयते प्रकाशावरणम् ।

52. tataH kshiiyate prakaashaavaraNaM

५३. धारणासु च योग्यता मनसः ।

53. dhaaraNaasu cha yogyataa manasaH

५४. स्वविषयासंप्रयोगे चित्तस्वरूपानुकार इवेन्द्रियाणां प्रत्याहारः ।

54. svavishhayaasa.nprayoge chittasvaruupaanukaara ive.ndriyaaNaaM pratyaahaaraH

५५. ततः परमा वश्यतेन्द्रियाणाम् ।

55.tataH paramaa vashyate.ndriyaaNaaM

इति श्रीपातञ्जले योगशास्त्रे साधननिर्देशो नाम द्वितीयः पादः ।

iti shriipaataJNjale yogashaastre saadhananirdesho naama dvitiiyaH paadaH

ॐ शान्तिश्शान्तिश्शान्तिः ।

OM shaa.ntishshaa.ntishshaa.ntiH

अथ श्रीपातञ्जलयोगदर्शनम् - विभूतिपादः ।

atha shriipaataJNjalayogadarshanaM vibhuutipaadaH

१. देशबन्धश्चित्तस्य धारणा ।

1. deshaba.ndhashchittasya dhaaraNaa

२. तत्र प्रत्ययैकतानता ध्यानम् ।

2. tatra pratyayaikataanataa dhyaanaM

३. तदेवार्थमात्रनिर्भासं स्वरूपशून्यमिव समाधिः ।

3. tadevaarthamaatranirbhaasaM svaruupashuunyamiva samaadhiH

४. त्रयमेकत्र संयमः ।

4. trayamekatra sa.nyamaH

५. तज्जयात्प्रज्ञाऽलोकः ।

5. tajjayaatpradnyaa.alokaH

६. तस्य भूमिषु विनियोगः ।

6. tasya bhuumishhu viniyogaH

७. त्रयमन्तरङ्गं पूर्वेभ्यः ।

7. trayama.ntara.ngaM puurvebhyaH

८. तदपि बहिरङ्गं निर्बीजस्य ।

8. tadapi bahira.ngaM nirbiijasya

९. व्युत्थाननिरोधसंस्कारयोरभिभवप्रादुर्भावौ निरोधक्षणचित्तान्वयो निरोधपरिणामः ।

9. vyutthaananirodhasa.nskaarayorabhibhavapraadurbhaavau nirodhakshaNachittaanvayo nirodhapariNaamaH

१०. तस्य प्रशान्तवाहिता संस्कारात् ।

10. tasya prashaa.ntavaahitaa sa.nskaaraat

११. सर्वार्थतैकाग्रतयोः क्षयोदयौ चित्तस्य समाधिपरिणामः ।

11. sarvaarthataikaagratayoH kshayodayau chittasya samaadhipariNaamaH

१२. शान्तोदितौ तुल्यप्रत्ययौ चित्तस्यैकाग्रतापरिणामः ।

12. shaa.ntoditau tulyapratyayau chittasyaikaagrataapariNaamaH

१३. एतेन भूतेन्द्रियेषु धर्मलक्षणावस्थापरिणामा व्याख्याताः ।

13. etena bhuute.ndriyeshhu dharmalakshaNaavasthaapariNaamaa vyaakhyaataaH

१४. शान्तोदिताव्यपदेश्यधर्मानुपाती धर्मी ।

14. shaa.ntoditaavyapadeshyadharmaanupaatii dharmii

१५. क्रमान्यत्वं परिणामान्यत्वे हेतुः ।

15. kramaanyatvaM pariNaamaanyatve hetuH

१६. परिणामत्रयसंयमादतीतानागतज्ञानम् ।

16. pariNaamatrayasa.nyamaadatiitaanaagatadnyaanaM

१७. शब्दार्थप्रत्ययानामितरेतराध्यासात् संकरस्तत्प्रविभागसंयमात्सर्वभूतरुतज्ञानम् ।

17. shabdaarthapratyayaanaamitaretaraadhyaasaat sa.nkarastatpravibhaagasa.nyamaatsarvabhuutaRutadnyaanaM

१८. संस्कारसाक्षात्करणात्पूर्वजातिज्ञानम् ।

18. sa.nskaarasaakshaatkaraNaatpuurvajaatidnyaanaM

१९. प्रत्ययस्य परचित्तज्ञानम् ।

19.pratyayasya parachittadnyaanaM

२०. न च तत्सालम्बनं तस्याविषयीभूतत्वात् ।

20. na cha tatsaalambanaM tasyaavishhayiibhuutatvaat

२१. कायरूपसंयमात्तद्ग्राह्यशक्तिस्तम्भे चक्षुःप्रकाशासंयोगेऽन्तर्धानम् ।

21. kaayaruupasa.nyamaattadgraahyashaktistambhe chakshuHprakaashaasa.nyoge.antardhaanaM

२२. सोपक्रमं निरुपक्रमं च कर्म तत्संयमादपरान्तज्ञानमरिष्टेभ्यो वा ।

22. sopakramaM nirupakramaM cha karma tatsa.nyamaadaparaa.ntadnyaanamarishhTebhyo vaa

२३. मैत्र्यादिषु बलानि ।

23. maitryaadishhu balaani

२४. बलेषु हस्तिबलादीनि ।

24. baleshhu hastibalaadiini

२५. प्रवृत्त्यालोकन्यासात्सूक्ष्मव्यवहितविप्रकृष्टज्ञानम् ।

25. pravRuttyaalokanyaasaatsuukshmavyavahitaviprakRushhTadnyaanaM

२६. भुवनज्ञानं सूर्ये संयमात् ।

26. bhuvanadnyaanaM suurye sa.nyamaat

२७. चन्द्रे ताराव्यूहज्ञानम् ।

27. cha.ndre taaraavyuuhadnyaanaM

२८. ध्रुवे तद्गतिज्ञानम् ।

28. dhruve tadgatidnyaanaM

२९. नाभिचक्रे कायव्यूहज्ञानम् ।

29. naabhichakre kaayavyuuhadnyaanaM

३०. कण्ठकूपे क्षुत्पिपासानिवृत्तिः ।

30. kaNThakuupe kshutpipaasaanivRuttiH

३१. कूर्मनाड्यां स्थैर्यम् ।

31. kuurmanaaDyaaM sthairyaM

३२. मूर्धज्योतिषि सिद्धदर्शनम् ।

32. muurdhajyotishhi siddhadarshanaM

३३. प्रातिभाद्वा सर्वम् ।

33. praatibhaadvaa sarvaM

३४. हृदये चित्तसंवित् ।

34. hRudaye chittasa.nvit

३५. सत्त्वपुरुषयोरत्यन्तासंकीर्णयोः प्रत्ययाविशेषो भोगः परार्थत्वात्स्वार्थसंयमात्पुरुषज्ञानम् ।

35. sattvapurushhayoratya.ntaasa.nkiirNayoH pratyayaavisheshho bhogaH paraarthatvaatsvaarthasa.nyamaatpurushhadnyaanaM

३६. ततः प्रातिभश्रावणवेदनादर्शास्वादवार्ता जायन्ते ।

36. tataH praatibhashraavaNavedanaadarshaasvaadavaartaa jaayante

३७. ते समाधावुपसर्गा व्युत्थाने सिद्धयः ।

37. te samaadhaavupasargaa vyutthaane siddhayaH

३८. बन्धकारणशैथिल्यात्प्रचारसंवेदनाच्च चित्तस्य परशरीरावेशः ।

38. ba.ndhakaaraNashaithilyaatprachaarasa.nvedanaachcha chittasya parashariiraaveshaH

३९. उदानजयाज्जलपङ्ककण्टकादिष्वसङ्ग उत्क्रान्तिश्च ।

39. udaanajayaajjalapa.nkakaNTakaadishhvasa.nga utkraantishcha

४०. समानजयाज्ज्वलनम् ।

40. samaanajayaajjvalanaM

४१. श्रोत्राकाशयोः संबन्धसंयमादिव्यं श्रोत्रम् ।

41. shrotraakaashayoH samba.ndhasa.nyamaaddivyaM shrotraM

४२. कायाकाशयोः संबन्धसंयमाल्लघुतूलसमापत्तेश्चाकाशगमनम् ।

42. kaayaakaashayoH samba.ndhasa.nyamaal-laghutuulasamaapatteshchaakaashagamanaM

४३. बहिरकल्पिता वृत्तिर्महाविदेहा ततः प्रकाशावरणक्षयः ।

43. bahirakalpitaa vRuttirmahaavidehaa tataH prakaashaavaraNakshayaH

४४. स्थूलस्वरूपसूक्ष्मान्वयार्थवत्त्वसंयमाद्भूतजयः ।

44. sthuulasvaruupasuukshmaanvayaarthavatvasa.nyamaadbhuutajayaH

४५. ततोऽणिमादिप्रादुर्भावः कायसंपत्तद्धर्मानभिघातश्च ।

45. tato.aNimaadipraadurbhaavaH kaayasampattaddharmaanabhighaatashcha

४६. रूपलावण्यबलवज्रसंहननत्वानि कायसंपत् ।

46. ruupalaavaNyabalavajrasa.nhananatvaani kaayasampat

४७. ग्रहणस्वरूपास्मितान्वयार्थवत्त्वसंयमादिन्द्रियजयः ।

47. grahaNasvaruupaasmitaanvayaarthavatvasa.nyamaadi.ndriyajayaH

४८. ततो मनोजवित्वं विकरणभावः प्रधानजयश्च ।

48. tato manojavitvaM vikaraNabhaavaH pradhaanajayashcha

४९. सत्त्वपुरुषान्यताख्यातिमात्रस्य सर्वभावाधिष्ठातृत्वं सर्वज्ञातृत्वं च ।

49. sattvapurushhaanyataakhyaatimaatrasya sarvabhaavaadhishhThaatRutvaM sarvadnyaatRutvaM cha

५०. तद्वैराग्यादपि दोषबीजक्षये कैवल्यम् ।

50. tadvairaagyaadapi doshhabiijakshaye kaivalyaM

५१. स्थान्युपनिमन्त्रणे सङ्गस्मयाकरणं पुनरनिष्टप्रसङ्गात् ।

51. sthaanyupanima.ntraNe sa.ngasmayaakaraNaM punaranishhTaprasa.ngaat

५२. क्षणतत्क्रमयोः संयमाद्विवेकजं ज्ञानम् ।

52. kshaNatatkramayoH sa.nyamaadvivekajaM dnyaanaM

५३. जातिलक्षणदेशैरन्यतानवच्छेदात् तुल्ययोस्ततः प्रतिपत्तिः ।

53. jaatilakshaNadeshairanyataanavachchhedaat tulyayostataH pratipattiH

५४. तारकं सर्वविषयं सर्वथाविषयमक्रमं चेति विवेकजं ज्ञानम् ।

54. taarakaM sarvavishhayaM sarvathaavishhayamakramaM cheti vivekajaM dnyaanaM

५५. सत्त्वपुरुषयोः शुद्धिसाम्ये कैवल्यम् ।

55. sattvapurushhayoH shuddhisaamye kaivalyaM

इति श्रीपातञ्जले योगशास्त्रे विभूतिनिर्देशो नाम तृतीयः पादः ।

iti shriipaataJNjale yogashaastre vibhuutinirdesho naama tRutiiyaH paadaH

ॐ शान्तिश्शान्तिश्शान्तिः ।

OM shaa.ntishshaa.ntishshaa.ntiH

अथ श्रीपातञ्जलयोगदर्शनम् - कैवल्यपादः ।

atha shriipaataJNjalayogadarshanaM kaivalyapaadaH

१. जन्मौषधिमन्त्रतपःसमाधिजाः सिद्धयः ।

1. janmaushhadhima.ntratapassamaadhijaaH siddhayaH

२. जात्यन्तरपरिणामः प्रकृत्यापूरात् ।

2. jaatya.ntarapariNaamaH prakRutyaapuuraat

३. निमित्तमप्रयोजकं प्रकृतीनां वरणभेदस्तु ततः क्षेत्रिकवत् ।

3. nimittamaprayojakaM prakRutiinaaM varaNabhedastu tataH kshetrikavat

४. निर्माणचित्तान्यस्मितामात्रात् ।

4. nirmaaNachittaanyasmitaamaatraat

५. प्रवृत्तिभेदे प्रयोजकं चित्तमेकमनेकेषाम् ।

5. pravRuttibhede prayojakaM chittamekamanekeshhaaM

६. तत्र ध्यानजमनाशयम् ।

6. tatra dhyaanajamanaashayaM

७. कर्माशुक्लाकृष्णं योगिनस्त्रिविधमितरेषाम् ।

7. karmaashuklaakRushhNaM yoginastrividhamitareshhaaM

८. ततस्तद्विपाकानुगुणानामेवाभिव्यक्तिर्वासनानाम् ।

8. tatastadvipaakaanuguNaanaamevaabhivyaktirvaasanaanaaM

९. जातिदेशकालव्यवहितानामप्यानन्तर्यं स्मृतिसंस्कारयोरेकरूपत्वात् ।

9. jaatideshakaalavyavahitaanaamapyaana.ntaryaM smRutisa.nskaarayorekaruupatvaat

१०. तासामनादित्वं चाशिषो नित्यत्वात् ।

10. taasaamanaaditvaM chaashishho nityatvaat

११. हेतुफलाश्रयालम्बनैः संगृहीतत्वादेषामभावे तदभावः ।

11. hetuphalaashrayaalambanaiH sa.ngRuhiitatvaadeshhaamabhaave tadabhaavaH

१२. अतीतानागतं स्वरूपतोऽस्त्यध्वभेदाद्धर्माणाम् ।

12. atiitaanaagataM svaruupato.astyadhvabhedaaddharmaaNaaM

१३. ते व्यक्तसूक्ष्मा गुणात्मानः ।

13. te vyaktasuukshmaa guNaatmaanaH

१४. परिणामैकत्वाद्वस्तुतत्त्वम् ।

14. pariNaamaikatvaadvastutattvaM

१५. वस्तुसाम्ये चित्तभेदात्तयोर्विभक्ताः पन्थाः ।

15. vastusaamye chittabhedaattayorvibhaktaaH panthaaH

१६. न चैकचित्ततन्त्रं वस्तु तदप्रमाणकं तदा किं स्यात् ।

16. na chaikachittata.ntraM vastu tadapramaaNakaM tadaa kiM syaat

१७. तदुपरागापेक्षित्वाच्चित्तस्य वस्तु ज्ञाताज्ञातम् ।

17. taduparaagaapekshitvaachchittasya vastu dnyaataadnyaataM

१८. सदा ज्ञाताश्चित्तवृत्तयस्तत्प्रभोः पुरुषस्यापरिणामित्वात् ।

18. sadaa dnyaataashchittavRuttayastatprabhoH purushhasyaapariNaamitvaat

१९. न तत्स्वाभासं दृश्यत्वात् ।

19. na tatsvaabhaasaM dRushyatvaat

२०. एकसमये चोभयानवधारणम् ।

20. ekasamaye chobhayaanavadhaaraNaM

२१. चित्तान्तरदृश्ये बुद्धिबुद्धेरतिप्रसङ्गः स्मृतिसंकरश्च ।

21. chittaa.ntaradRushye buddhibuddheratiprasa.ngaH smRutisa.nkarashcha

२२. चितेरप्रतिसंक्रमायास्तदाकारापत्तौ स्वबुद्धिसंवेदनम् ।

22. chiterapratisa.nkramaayaastadaakaaraapattau svabuddhisa.nvedanaM

२३. द्रष्टृदृश्योपरक्तं चित्तं सर्वार्थम् ।

23. drashhTRudRushyoparaktaM chittaM sarvaarthaM

२४. तदसंख्येयवासनाभिश्चित्रमपि परार्थं संहत्यकारित्वात् ।

24. tadasa.nkhyeyavaasanaabhishchitramapi paraarthaM sa.nhatyakaaritvaat

२५. विशेषदर्शिन आत्मभावभावनाविनिवृत्तिः ।

25. visheshhadarshina aatmabhaavabhaavanaavinivRuttiH

२६. तदा विवेकनिम्नं कैवल्यप्राग्भारं चित्तम् ।

26. tadaa vivekanimnaM kaivalyapraagbhaaraM chittaM

२७. तच्छिद्रेषु प्रत्ययान्तराणि संस्कारेभ्यः ।

27. tachchhidreshhu pratyayaa.ntaraaNi sa.nskaarebhyaH

२८. हानमेषां क्लेशवदुक्तम् ।

28. haanameshhaaM kleshavaduktaM

२९. प्रसंख्यानेऽप्यकुसीदस्य सर्वथा विवेकख्यातेर्धर्ममेघः समाधिः ।

29. prasa.nkhyaane.apyakusiidasya sarvathaa vivekakhyaaterdharmamegha-ssamaadhiH

३०. ततः क्लेशकर्मनिवृत्तिः ।

30. tataH kleshakarmanivRuttiH

३१. तदा सर्वावरणमलापेतस्य ज्ञानस्याऽनन्त्याज्ज्ञेयमल्पम् ।

31. tadaa sarvaavaraNamalaapetasya dnyaanasyaa.ana.ntyaajdnyeyaM alpaM

३२. ततः कृतार्थानां परिणामक्रमसमाप्तिर्गुणानाम् ।

32. tataH kRutaarthaanaaM pariNaamakramasamaaptirguNaanaaM

३३. क्षणप्रतियोगी परिणामापरान्तनिर्ग्राह्यः क्रमः ।

33. kshaNapratiyogii pariNaamaaparaa.ntanirgraahyaH kramaH

३४. पुरुषार्थशून्यानां गुणानां प्रतिप्रसवः कैवल्यं स्वरूपप्रतिष्ठा वा चितिशक्तिरिति ।

34. purushhaarthashuunyaanaaM guNaanaaM pratiprasavaH kaivalyaM svaruupapratishhThaa vaa chitishaktiriti

इति श्रीपातञ्जले योगशास्त्रे कैवल्यनिरूपणं नाम चतुर्थः पादः ।

iti shriipaataJNjale yogashaastre kaivalyaniruupaNaM naama chaturthaH paadaH

॥ समाप्तं योगदर्शनम् ॥

samaaptaM yogadarshanaM

ॐ शान्तिश्शान्तिश्शान्तिः ।

OM shaa.ntishshaa.ntishshaa.ntiH

<u>Student Notes</u>

वन्दना (Prayer)

(योगदर्शन प्रणेतारं महर्षि-पतञ्जलिं प्रति सादरं वन्दना ।)

(श्लोक: - वसन्ततिलकावृत्तम्)

चेतोवृपुर्विकसनाय सदा समेषाम्

अष्टाङ्गयोगमिह य: कथयाञ्चकार ।

येनोज्ज्वलोऽन्धतमसे विदधे सुपन्था

वन्दे पतञ्जलि-मुनिं करुणाकरं तम् ॥

गीतम् (Song)

येन दर्शितो येन बोधितो सन्मार्गो जगते ।

भगवान् पतञ्जलिर्वन्द्यते ॥धृ.॥

यमनियमप्रभृतीन्यङ्गानि

येनाष्टौ संप्रकीर्तितानि

मनुजानां कल्याणसंततिं निरन्तरं तन्वते ॥१॥

शरीरमाद्यं धर्मसाधनं

प्रभुणा दत्तं महन्निधानं

येनोपायस्तद्रक्षार्थं शास्त्रे प्रविधीयते ॥२॥

चेतोवृत्तिनिरोधो योग:

तत्सामर्थ्यान्नश्यति रोग:

सबलशरीरे सबलमानसं येनैवं कथ्यते ॥३॥

योग: कर्मसु कौशलमेवं

भगवद्गीता कथयति भावं

येनार्थोदयं योगदर्शने प्रत्यक्षी क्रियते ॥४॥

अष्टगुणोऽयं योगदीपक:

तेनोज्ज्वलित: सकलो लोक:

भुवि प्रकाशस्तस्य हितकर: सनातनो राजते ॥५॥

नमो नमो भगवते योगिने

नमो जगत्कल्याणकारिणे

नमो महर्षे पतञ्जलेऽयं कराञ्जलिर्बध्यते ॥६॥

(Composition by Dr. Deviprasad Kharwandikar)

Yoga Instruction Materials

- **Yoga Exercise Instructional Videos:**
  o Soorya Namaskar (Sun Salutations) Level I
  o Soorya Namaskar (Sun Salutations) Level II (advanced)
  o Authenticy Yoga Level I

- **Yoga Exercise Instructional Audios:**
  o Authentic Yoga Meditation Course
  o Authentic Yoga Level I

- **Books and Audios:**
  o Yoga Sutras of Patanjali - Proper Translation & Chanting
  o Health and Yoga Aphorisms of SaeeTech The Authentic Yoga School, Copyright SaeeTech, available in many languages
  o Shree Ganesha Atharvasheersham Guided Recitation, English Translation and Comprehensive Explanation
  o Shree Ramaraksha Stotra Mantram Guided Recitation, English Translation and Comprehensive Explanation
  o Guide to Spiritual Life
  o Health and Yoga Aphorisms of SaeeTech with English Commentary and Sanskrit Version Verses and Sanskrit Chanting Audio

- **Seminar Videos and Audios:**
  o Yoga Sutras of Patanjali - explanatory speeches (17 videos)
  o Health Part I and Part II
  o Nutrition Part I, Part II, and Part III
  o Correct Weight Management
  o Correct Stress Management Part I and Part II
  o Speeches on various Yoga Topics

- **Chanting Audios:**
  o Shree Ganesha Atharvasheersham
  o Shree Ramaraksha Stotra Mantram
  o Shree Sooryanamaskar
  o Shree Gangalahari
  o Shree Gayatri and Mahamritinjaya mantrams
  o Shree Ganesha and Vishnu Sahasranama
  o Yoga Sutras of Patanjali - Normal chanting & Guided instruction

---

Please refer to the website **www.authenticyoga.org** for additional details.

May the entire creation be filled with peace and joy. **OM Shaantih.**